The Body
in Recovery

The Body
in Recovery

Somatic Psychotherapy and the Self

John P. Conger

Frog, Ltd.
Berkeley, California

Notice to the Reader

This book is not intended to replace good medical diagnosis and treatment. Its purpose is to help you work with your health care practitioner in making informed treatment decisions.

The Body in Recovery: Somatic Psychotherapy and the Self

Published by
Frog, Ltd.

Frog, Ltd. books are distributed by
North Atlantic Books
P.O. Box 12327
Berkeley, California 94701

Cover and book design by Paula Morrison
Typeset by Catherine Campaigne
Printed in the United States of America by Malloy Lithographing

First Frog, Ltd. publication 1994

Library of Congress Cataloging-in-Publication Data

Conger, John P., 1935–
    The body in recovery : somatic psychotherapy and the self / John
P. Conger.
    p. cm.
    ISBN 1–883319–06–4
    1. Mind and body therapies.   2. Bioenergetic psychotherapy.
    I. Title.
    RC489.M53C66 1993
    616.89'14—dc20   93–37231
                                                                       CIP

1 2 3 4 5 6 7 8 9 / 98 97 96 95 94

This book is gratefully dedicated to my three sons,
Tim, Gregory, and Rhys.

Acknowledgments

I wish to thank my wife for her support and encouragement during the writing of this book. She was not only a devoted and wonderful friend but an excellent editor, whose words often filled the gaps in my thought. I thank my son Tim who typed the barely legible early manuscript, and encouraged me to continue.

I wish to thank Eleanor Greenlee, a trainer in Bioenergetics, whose exceptional gifts at reading the body became a model out of which my work proceeds. I also owe a debt of gratitude to the Bioenergetic community for training, professional discussion, and fellowship, and to Myron Sharaf for his breadth of understanding, his critical intelligence, his humor and his friendship.

I am also deeply grateful to my friends for reading the manuscript during its evolution. I have been most fortunate to have their learned reflections, enthusiastic support and their candid criticism, which allowed me to make extensive revisions. In particular, I thank Peter Bernhardt, Mike Hansen, Howard Treibitz, Scott Baum, Marvin Spiegelman, Michael Conant, Susan Merrill, Sue von Baeyer, Maryanna Eckberg, Helen Resneck, Steve Galper and Judith Bell.

If your life has not three dimensions, if you don't live in the body, if you live on the two dimensional plane in the paper world that is flat and printed, as if you were only living your biography, then you are nowhere. You don't see the archetypal world, but live like a pressed flower in the pages of a book, a mere memory of yourself.

C. G. Jung, *Nietzsche's Zarathustra*

Contents

A List of Exercises

Introduction

> If the doors of perception were cleansed everything would appear to man as it is, infinite. For man has closed himself up, till he sees all things thro' narrow chinks of his cavern.
>
> William Blake, "A Memorable Fancy."

To the early followers of Freud, psychoanalysis was a stunning revolution transforming their vision of human nature. Their eyes were opened. They saw neurosis as epidemic in proportion. They saw humanity in the grip of unconscious forces, men and women imagining a freedom of choice that was not, in reality, theirs. Like Plato's vision, people were chained in a dark cave staring at shadows on a wall cast by a flickering fire, unable and unwilling to pass through the cave's mouth into the full light of day.

A brilliant young student of Freud's in the 1920s, Wilhelm Reich, carried on the revolution through his investigation of character, genitality and body armoring. In his study of the effect of muscular contraction on energetic flow, Reich gave us practical techniques to transform our dark body home.

Through a psychological body therapy, our eyes have been opened. Revealed to us now, we see the body, in need of recovery, treated as a possession separate from ourselves. Many of us have lived like renters in a small room of a house we consider barely habitable. Disembodied, we have dangerously compromised the fabric of nature that supports us. We have come to see that on our fragile planet, we must become accountable to our body as well as our mind and spirit.

We may be wrong when we blame aging alone for our loss of function and feeling. Sometimes areas of our body become gray and lifeless. We lose our vitality and our hunger for life. We pin all our hopes on diets. We suffer from chronic physical problems, problems with our backs, our stomachs, our feet, and our frequent solution becomes pain killers. Our illnesses may not be inevitable. A powerful remnant of our past lies anchored in body structure "unrecovered," creating pockets of weakness open in time to illness and strain. Our bodies will for years carry the burden of unhealed injuries. Many people do not know how to work through the losses life brings. Our body faithfully records the traumatic events in contracted musculature and energetically withdrawn tissue.

When we no longer experience pleasure in our bodies in the ordinary tasks of life, we build patterns to deny the body altogether. We don't even walk for exercise. We prefer our bodies to keep silent so that we can conduct our life undisturbed in our psyche. Through a psychological body therapy we can restore feeling and pleasure in our bodily and emotional expression. We need not suffer in a body prison. We can be more liberated and embodied. Unfortunately optimistic promises are cheap and change comes at a high price. Embodiment means giving up illusion, grandiosity, specialness for the sake of an honest grounded reality, genuine contact and relatedness and pleasure in the basic experiences of life.

This book presents step-by-step instructions along a path toward the body's recovery from the trauma accumulated through the years of a "normal" life. Intended as a guide for therapists, clients and other interested people, this book discusses psychological and somatic (body-oriented) principles and concepts essential to a responsible psychologically oriented body therapy. Practical exercises develop kinesthetic awareness and access suppressed emotional states. In recovery we become grounded and develop clear boundaries. We search out our vital nature and throw off the body's overcoat of fearful and angry constraint. In developing a functional and durable self, we rediscover the pleasure in the ordinary movements of daily life.

Although we tend to separate the body and psyche in our daily lives, they are united through an inner self which appears to direct us. We are lived by this inner self. In our therapy we try to understand the directing inner self and effect a healthy outcome through bodywork and interpretation. A carpenter, referred to me by a chiropractor, had been told by several doctors that his lower back revealed genetic defects that would remain unstable unless some discs were fused. Even with this radical procedure he was going to have difficulties for the rest of his life. The diagnosis did not explain his physically free-wheeling life style up until that point. Refusing surgery the client was bed-ridden and in pain for months while getting up for basic self care and to attend chiropractic and psychotherapy appointments. He slowly got in touch with his inner nature that expresses itself through psyche and soma. He began to listen for the meaning of the pain and to choose less hurtful directions for his life. Gradually his back healed. He changed professions. Now his back occasionally warns him through discomfort against an unhealthy direction. Other clients, too, have become grateful to their sensitive backs.

A psychological body therapy is a powerful medium that awakens unconscious images and energy and calls for therapeutic assistance. The isolated style of the romantic hero, facing difficulties alone, has not proven successful in the shadows of the self where courage is measured by speaking the truth about ourselves to others. Disclosures of our humanity are both miraculous and commonplace. On the one hand we do not need experts, coveting knowledge as power, to lead us to our nature, rattling the bones of revelation in our upturned incredulous faces. We can read the information for ourselves about incest, relationships, sexual intimacy, the injuries of childhood and the mysteries of body structure. On the other hand a psychologically-oriented body therapy utilizes powerful techniques which demand experienced therapists to guide us.

There have been two paths in body therapy. In the first path the focus has been to identify and confront the defense structure or "character" as Reich called it, to unblock the body structure so that the body's healthy rhythms can awaken or reassert themselves. In the second path, supportive attention calls forth the hidden resources of healthy functioning to throw off the body's unnecessary encumbrances. Following either path the therapist needs to see the client in his or her uniqueness, and facilitate a deepening dialogue with the inner self. It is this inner self that understands the meaning and direction of our health and illness.

Experienced body therapists are likely to be both confrontive and supportive, active and still, according to therapeutic necessity. Yet the different body therapies arrange their techniques to emphasize one approach or the other. While my intention has been to be inclusive, this book reflects my general preference for the first path. In this book we study and identify character, and use exercises to loosen rigidities in body structure, but we also support gentle techniques in which the therapist is witness to the subtle energetic pulsation transmitting itself throughout the undeveloped body areas. In silence our hands speak fluently in the language of the body.

Wilhelm Reich, the grandfather of my approach, tenaciously held to a biological model in his therapeutic work. He argued that all neurosis was caused by the damming up of libidinal energy and that psychic conflict alone was not sufficiently disruptive to cause illness. Initially Reich was merely expanding the claims of Freud's earlier conclusion which stated that some neurosis was caused by the damming up of libido. Reich came to understand in the 1930's that repressed instinctual energy experienced as anxiety was diminished and made tolerable through character armor, a body response involving the chronic contractions of muscle groups. When the body felt a full sexual orgasm, it was able to clear itself of unreleased energies. Thus, Reich worked to resolve blocks to the flow of energy so that a full release was possible.

Since Reich's death in 1957, many practitioners have expanded the knowledge and techniques of body therapy. They have stepped past the single focus on genital release, while acknowledging its preeminence. For instance, Dr Trygve Braatoy and Ms Aadel Bulow-Hansen, working with patients in Oslo, Norway, developed a body psycho-analysis and training that influenced Lillemor Johnsen and Gerda Boyesen. In contrast to Reich's fascination with hypertonic muscle (very tense), Lillemor Johnsen brought our attention to the undeveloped musculature, the hypotonic (slack) muscle that held repressed energies and the deep resources of an emerging self. She has used different colors to map the body tonus, and has worked with the pulsations of breath that move in waves through the body.

Gerda Boyesen has worked with the release of visceral holding.

Lisbeth Marcher has refined Johnsen's body map to evaluate the tension or slackness of specific muscles, in order to restore healthy tonus and balance to the body. Because individual muscles begin functioning in accordance with a developmental time frame, muscular tonus reflects trauma at specific childhood periods. Influenced by Frank Lake's discussion of an intra-uterine psychology in *Clinical Theology* (London: 1966), Marcher developed seven character positions.

Inspired by his teacher Wilhelm Reich, Alexander Lowen delineated the psychological and physical characteristics of five character structures related to childhood development. Working with the body standing up as well as lying down, Lowen created techniques to disrupt body armor and release repressed emotion, promoting a more graceful and alive bodily expression.

Another student of Reich's, Myron Sharaf, who wrote the definitive biography of Reich, *Fury On Earth,* has continued through the years to explore, in writing, teaching and private practice, the relationship of Reichian psychotherapy to psychoanalysis. A thoughtful, gifted therapist, he has represented an inclusive Reichian perspective rich in humanity and intelligence. David Boadella, through his books, his private practice and his journal, *Energy and Character,* has furthered research and understanding in somatic therapy, practice and theory. Stanley Keleman, in eloquent books, has explored the biological metaphor and the fundamentals of our embodied life. And of course, there are other clinicians and theorists, too numerous to mention, who have brought somatic work to a richer place.

Unfortunately a psychologically-oriented body therapy has not always been understood or accepted by practitioners of other psychological disciplines. Theoretical differences are partly responsible; also somaticists have failed to explain themselves in terms other disciplines can value. To some degree insularity, egocentricity, self-interest and competitiveness have kept the entire psychological community at war with each other, representing a failure in vision and humanity.

There is a history to some of our theoretical differences. In the 1920s, Reich found himself reluctantly at odds on several issues with his hero and mentor, Sigmund Freud. Reich found that patients often were uneffected by powerful interpretations aimed at revealing the psychological underpinnings of their neurosis. Through a partially hidden attitude, the patient was able to resist the impact of insight. A smile of superiority or a hostile joke about therapy were clues to a character resistance that Reich insisted must be confronted before interpretations were made. Freud insisted that interpretations of psychological material be made as soon as they appeared in the therapy. Psychoanalytic practice has come to agree with Reich's position in this matter. This confrontation of character attitude became a foundation of Reichian body therapy.

In the 1890s, Freud's patients described how in childhood, family members had sexually molested them, in particular, the father. Supporting the truth of these claims, Freud often found that the therapy foundered. In 1897 Freud abandoned his Seduction Theory. His self-analysis led him instead to an understanding of sexual fantasy in children and the Oedipal Complex. Freud shifted from an interpersonal to intrapsychic theory. According to his revised theory, the inner world of sexual instincts and fantasy was in conflict with the outer world of culture. The repression of instinctual drives caused illness. Reich remained a passionate believer in this Topographical Theory, as it was called.

In the early 1920s, Freud postulated a death instinct which he thought explained many therapeutic failures. Reich disagreed with Freud's latest radical speculation and with his new Structural Theory that described a largely unconscious super-ego in conflict with id impulses while a mediating ego with limited powers looked on. With this theoretical leap, psychoanalysis became an entirely intrapsychic system. In a new framework psychoanalysis would be unable to accept or understand a body-oriented psychotherapy with an interpersonal as well as an intrapsychic base. Years later Heinz Kohut was to come to a similar impasse with psychoanalytic theory, which led to the development of Self Psychology, a discipline that acknowledges the necessity of an interpersonal component.

Each new psychological system reaches out to solve all of human suffering. In the early days body therapists were tempted to exalt the body as the sole answer to psychological health. The euphoria over a body heaven has suffered disillusion of a failed dream, another attempt to claim exclusive rights to life's mystery. Psychology has developed technically and theoretically since the 1920s, and so must an inclusive body therapy evolve into a more sophisticated enterprise or be relegated forever to a rebellious counter culture. If this powerful therapeutic discipline is to place itself centrally, it must come to terms with a psychology of the self as well as a psychology of instinctual repression and find support in both intrapsychic and interpersonal theory. For theory and somatic wisdom, this book gratefully acknowledges a debt to the work of Sigmund Freud, Carl Jung, Georg Groddeck, Sandor Ferenczi, Melanie Klein, W.R.D. Fairbairn, D. W. Winnicott, M. Masud R. Khan, Harold F. Searles, Heinz Kohut, Wilhelm Reich, Lillemor Johnsen, Gerda Boyesen, Lisbeth Marcher, David Boadella, Ida Rolf, Moshe Feldenkrais, Stanley Keleman, Myron Sharaf and Alexander Lowen. I am committed to a model of body therapy informed and enlarged by psychodynamic theory.

The first section of the book, ***The Therapist and Transference,*** discusses issues relevant to students of body therapy. There are essays on touch and transference, useful equipment, reading body energy, the tools of body therapy, and initial professional procedures. The next four sections provide a progressive series of concepts and exercises that typically might be carried through in a psychological body analysis.

Section Two, ***Contact and Kinesthetic Awareness,*** explores five principles that promote contact: grounding, good boundaries, unrestricted breathing, access to emotion and intention. To be in contact is to be fully present here and now.

We identify and disarm character and differentiate ourselves psychologically and physically from our family members in the next section, ***Character and Restructuring.*** Alexander Lowen's five character types are described. We work on restructuring through attention to eight stations of the body-standing-up.

In Section Four, *Protest and Emotional Expression,* we seek to recover our energetic expression and liberate our emotional life. The suppression of our nature has taken place at the cost of our capacity to protest, to stand up for ourselves. We work with Reich's seven segments and the body-lying-down.

The fifth section, *Embodiment and the Psyche-Soma Correspondence,* addresses the development of self through relatedness and through the healing of splits. We explore six basic body divisions. It is not enough to crash through the body's repressive wall to liberate lost feeling and energy. If we have failed to develop physically and emotionally, we have also failed to call forth our potential nature and to integrate the lost aspects of self.

While I owe a debt to the many theorists and friends who deepened my psychological awareness and to my extensive training in Bioenergetics, of which I proudly remain a trainer, there are aspects of this book that originate with my own work with clients: the seven tools of a psychological body therapy, the five principles of contact, the eight stations of the body-standing-up, the six basic body divisions, the three body signatures, the divisions of space, the shadow and ideal body, some of the exercises, the integration of theory with subtle aspects of presentation and thought.

This book is the culmination of many years of personal and professional development. I am no longer young, and age has only intensified my appreciation and passion for this work. What is the point of living bent over if we need not do so? What does it mean spiritually and psychologically to be physically ungrounded, or walk with a pelvis that does not move, or talk from a head that seems suspended incongruously above the ground, the assisting body a stuffed bear? What recourse is there when our sexual life is unfulfilling? Quite marvelously a psychologically-oriented body therapy can help us. Many people, in the grip of intense spiritual longing, have attempted to separate themselves from the physical world, only to discover that spiritual progress depends on transformation through embodiment. You can lift spiritually with more ease when you stand firmly on the ground. Somatic recovery leads to wholeness and the simplicity of embodied life.

Section One

The Therapist
and Transference

Chapter 1

In Search of a Model for a Body-Oriented Psychotherapy

> When I am not cheerful and master of myself, every single one of my patients is a tormenting spirit to me.... I adopted the expedient of renouncing working by conscious thought, so as to grope my way further into the riddles only by blind touch. Since I started this I have been doing my work, perhaps more skilfully than before, but I do not know what I am doing.
>
> —S. Freud, Letter to Wilhelm Fliess, 1900

After the publication of his book on dreams, Freud endured painful disappointment. He did not experience the recognition and prosperity he had wished for. He hated Vienna, he said. With this seeming failure, Freud temporarily lost his taste for strategy in therapy. He dropped his professional personna and worked with clients by immediate felt response. Carl Jung had a similar period as he was breaking up with Freud in 1912. Jung also abandoned his professional mask and conducted therapy as if with no preconceptions. "I avoided all theoretical points of view and simply helped the patients to understand the dream-images by themselves...."[1] Both Freud and Jung reported positive results.

To meet the client in his or her uniqueness, we must let go of rigidly held assumptions or risk reducing the client to a shadowy player in our theoretical system. Insofar as we leave room for a sincere encounter, we have an interpersonal therapy. Our professional demeanor has value, but our basic humanity, honest questioning, our awareness of personal limitation and our grounded presence encourage the deepest change in our clients. Mental knowledge, so essential to the development of our work, must translate down to blood and muscle, to our capacity to be embodied. As Jung said, Freud healed people because he was a kind man.

As a researcher and doctor, Freud began with a biological model where touch was understood as a functional necessity. In the early years of psychoanalysis, Freud, in keeping with the scientific viewpoint of his old teacher and employer Ernst Bruche, attempted to explain psychological response solely in terms of neurophysiology. In the autumn of 1895, he sent his essay about this, known as "The Project," to his friend Fliess, and never reclaimed it. Freud gradually distanced himself from a biological approach to psychology and from his friend Fliess who had so challenged his mind in the past with biological surmises. Liberated from the parent discipline of biology, Freud developed rules and a conceptual structure of its own for psychology.

For many years Freud held to the toxicological theory of "actual neurosis" which argued that through faulty sexual practices of excessive masturbation or coitus interruptus, dammed up libido caused neurotic illness, a theory that inspired Reich in the 1920s. And yet with years of impressive research in neuroanatomy behind him, Freud developed a psychology more at home among the literary and philosophically minded than reductionistic biological scientists. When in 1897, Freud abandoned the seduction theory and replaced it with an intrapsychic model of repressed instinct and fantasy, he put the body to sleep. He had only himself in the room during his self analysis with his courageous dream book as a witness.

The medical community saw only the influence of the body on the mind of their patients but Freud argued that the relation between the body and mind was reciprocal. In 1905 in "Psychical (or Mental) Treatment" Freud stated, "The relation between body and mind (in animals no less than in human beings) is a reciprocal one; but in earlier times the other side of this relation, the effect of the mind upon the body, found little favour in the eyes of physicians."[2] He argued for the effect of strong, persistent, feeling on the body's disposition and health. He discussed illness traceable to the mind and the use of hypnosis. As a method of intervening in the psyche-soma relationship, Freud was in love with words rather than touch.

> Words are the most important media by which one man seeks to bring his influence to bear on another; words are a good method of producing mental changes in the person to whom they are addressed. So that there is no longer anything puzzling in the assertion that the magic of words can remove the symptoms of illness, and especially such as are themselves founded on mental states.[3]

In later years, Freud partially understood and partially rejected a therapy using touch. Freud did not interfere with Ferenczi who hugged and even kissed his clients in his active technique, but was horrified that Ferenczi might publish his findings. Exploring the somatic, the interpersonal and the intrapsychic dimensions of psychotherapy, Ferenczi struggled with techniques to assist clients with fragmented self structure. He tried to join with clients to be the glue to integrate painful memories. He utilized a play therapy with adults. He made himself vulnerable through mutual analysis, a technique therapists had practiced among themselves. When clients needed it, he mothered them. Such seriously disturbed clients would have otherwise been dismissed as unsuitable for psychoanalysis. Ferenczi, who was Melanie Klein's therapist in her early professional life, undoubtedly influenced her development of play therapy and had an impact on the work of other English Object Relations therapists.

Many years later Heinz Kohut, a recognized leader in psychoanalysis founded a self psychology based on an interpersonal and intrapsychic model. Improvements, he said, in some patients with a primary disorder of the self, took place through responses that the psychoanalyst considered peripheral. "In other words, I believe that appropriate responses to primary self pathology have in the past been given, at times reluctantly and even guiltily, by a number of intuitive analysts—with good results."[4]

Kohut believed that in narcissistic personality disorders, the self of the client was confirmed and made cohesive by appropriate responses of the mirroring and the idealized self-object. With this practice, instead of dismissing the idealizing transference, the therapist allows the client time to incorporate his idealized form as essential in the building of a functional self. From the perspective of Self Psychology we can understand Ferenczi's active technique which stood against the directives of an intrapsychic drive psychology. Kohut's supportive treatment of patients stands in contradiction to the neutrality advocated by classical psychoanalysis.

> One of the problems with traditional analysis is that it was—and continues to be—a clandestine moral system: Drives need to be tamed. People are born uncivilized and need to become civilized, and, alas, this is not fully doable or achievable. Nobody admits this is so, but it is implicit in the drive primacy theory.[5]

In contrast, Kohut says, his values are "to support human psychological life to its fullest."[6] When appropriate the therapist is supportive. A child who is not mirrored or given approval despairs. Hope "is absolutely needed for psychological survival."[7]

In its youth, psychoanalysis was more comprehensive concerned with being inclusive, notwithstanding its painful expulsions of Adler, Jung, Rank, Ferenczi and Reich. In the 1920s, when dual relationships abounded, Freud's clients became his analysts and he invited them to dinner and shared his library; during those early days, boundaries were blurred. Even with the prejudice against body, touch was another possibility for the future to be discreetly explored. But with time, psychoanalysis developed its own purity of style. Gone from the analysts office and waiting room were the antique statues, the personal gifts, books and pictures, and any objects that provided much clue to the real identity of the therapist, so that the projection screen might be clear.

In contrast, Freud, by moving behind the couch, had left profound evidence of himself through his many objects, as tokens of his ideal personal presence in the room. To the displaced Viennese psychoanalyst in exile, the empty office may have reflected the cultural impoverishment of the dreaded New World where as analysts they uncomfortably settled, missing the relaxed informality of the old Vienna. Freud's losing battle for a model of a non-medical psychoanalytic therapist underlined the defeat of a broad cultural understanding in favor of a preserving narrow science.

We cannot return to the days before Hitler which were far from ideal in any case, but perhaps we can catch a glimpse of the depth and breadth of psychoanalysis before it narrowed down. Donald Winnicott, an English pediatrician and analyst, seems to have been able to embrace psychoanalysis in a way that left him room to explore and theorize in relative freedom. He could explore a squiggle game and share drawing with his young clients. While child therapy is as disciplined as adult psychoanalysis, the rules of touching are mercifully different with children, because for children, touching is food. Touching is essential. We cannot persuade children otherwise as we can with adults.

Carl Jung, like Winnicott, was not dismissive of the body nor did he feel any obligation to be out of sight or clear his room of personal reference. Since his clients came from other countries, they were given opportunities to mix socially with each other rather than be alone away from home. Jung worked from an interpersonal model although he clearly preferred the intrapsychic elements in therapy. His alchemical model places the therapist "in the soup" with the client, subject to the profound forces of the unconscious.

While he warned against the illusion of objectivity by the therapist who wished to be removed from the client's process, Jung regarded the transference as a nuisance in the therapy. The personal aspect of therapy, the mother-father transference bored him. He sought out the archetypal elements, the dreams that related to those features of life that touched into the universal and mythic themes. Jung was a brilliant therapist. In one story about his work, a young woman was sent to him by a colleague from another country who could do nothing for her. In a single session, Jung held the client rocking her and singing nursery songs, a session that changed her life.

With the many remarkable models for a body-oriented psychotherapy, I find myself drawn back to Georg Groddeck, a friend and disciple of Freud. Groddeck was a physician who worked with clients utilizing massage, diet, psychoanalysis and the baths of Baden-Baden. Groddeck's *The Book of the It* and Freud's *The Ego and The Id* were published within months of each other in the first half of 1923. Although Freud partially derived his concept of the id from Groddeck, Groddeck did not accept Freud's reductionism to conscious and unconscious, ego and id, nor did Freud accept Groddeck's "It mythology."

For years Freud turned down Groddeck's requests to visit him at Baden-Baden where Ferenzci and Rank had visited, engaging in a mutual analysis. Even while recovering from cancer of the jaw operated on for the first time in the second half of 1923, Freud refused Groddeck's invitation. While Groddeck used psychoanalysis in working with his patients and enjoyed a protected "disciple" status until his death in 1934, he viewed Freud's healing process in an encompassing frame where cancer of the jaw was caused by more than smoking cigars. He explored illness as a doorway to the inner self.

Groddeck did not leave to us a complex structure of thought; he was not so much a theorist as a healer. His writing is impassioned rather than linear. Yet his inclusive model of healing using diet, massage, the baths and psychoanalysis along with his active dialogue with the It as the centerpiece of the system, is brilliant and effective. We sense in his writing his pragmatic, down-to-earth, unpretentious nature and his intuitive gifts. Jung explained an underlying presence that included body and psyche, but Groddeck gave us the experience through examples and self-report.

Unattractive as the term "It" is, his vision of the It is compelling for the somatic psychotherapist. Groddeck said that the body is held in the middle between polarities with a leaning toward the left or right, health or illness, male or femaleness. The It expresses

8

through sickness as well as health and we are never entirely sick or entirely well. We are not entirely male or female, strong or weak, intelligent or stupid, coordinated or uncoordinated. Our ego identity is but a small surface aspect of the organizing principle that encompasses our body, psyche and spirit. The It does not regard time, space, sex or age. Differences are blurred. The child speaks in the adult and the adult appears in the child. Like Jung's encompassing Self, the It, hold us in a balance of polarities.

> The It influences fat formation, growth and character as if it were a rational being. It is the duty of the doctor to find out what meaning this uncomfortable obesity may have, with its attendant dangers of a stroke, heart trouble, or dropsy, what this leanness and tuberculosis may signify. The unconscious does not merely reveal itself in dreams, it reveals itself in every gesture, in the twitching of the forehead, the beating of the heart, yet also in the quiet warning of a uric-acid diathesis.... [8]

Groddeck saw the It as sensitive and cautious, creating safe havens for itself. Illness can bring rest and protection from the outside world. When young, Groddeck himself suffered from an initially harmless wound on his knee. This later developed into a permanent weakness on his left side, causing physical realignment and a characterological shift toward reticence and away from hastiness.

> In the course of my later life I developed sciatica and gout troubles with deformities of the joints which for decades, temporarily and apparently never without reason and purpose, made it impossible for me to go for long walks and sometimes even prevented me from walking at all. In recent years this condition has improved decisively—I may be allowed to say only by applying self-analysis—and not only has the pain gone, but my toes, which once pointed sideways, have now reverted to the normal straight position. And yet I can still discover a curious interaction between the physical pain of gout and the cautious hesitation which makes me avoid or reduce physical danger, and I always deserve a special kind of enjoyment from this, such as one only gets from ironic observation of one's self. [9]

As therapists of a psychological bodywork, the conflict between Groddeck and Freud, between respected, long-term friends, has meaning. The narrowing focus of scientific endeavor in psychoanalysis has brought unique and irreplaceable results in the study of human nature. We can neither dismiss so profound a history nor abandon our own valid roots. Through the whole sweep of psychological study we can find knowledge of psyche-soma relationship and ground ourselves in the center of developing knowledge. But particularly we may want to anchor our ship in the harbors of Freud, Groddeck, Jung, Reich, Ferenczi, Winnicott, Kohut and Lowen because of an inclusive awareness of the blend of body, psyche and spirit.

Embodiment has to do with the blend of that central intelligence beyond mere ego that lives us and dreams us. We can cooperate and also intervene in the Self's expression where healing seems desirable. Sometimes illnesses are not to be cured because they fulfill purposes we cannot reach or understand. And yet illness as an expression may be replaced by the unconscious made conscious, by accessing a primitive underlying image that contracted us in terror in childhood. Embodiment is not perfect health but rather a consciousness of wholeness and relatedness, a standing in the center of many polarities as an inventive, curious presence in a state of spontaneous play.

Chapter 2

Transference and Touch

There are myriad forms of bodywork although few forms are psychologically oriented and therefore accountable to the implications of relationship and touching. For instance, we do not explore with our masseur the implications of touching. Nevertheless, we are profoundly affected by the conventions of that discipline which provides safe boundaries of expectation held unspoken in mutual agreement. If a benignly intended massage becomes sexual, we are profoundly violated. If a masseur or masseuse verbally interprets our structure to us uninvited, we are violated. All forms of bodywork are responsible to conventions particular to the individual form, and disregard of client boundaries need to be considered with the greatest seriousness. Ethically and practically, it is essential that all bodyworkers spell out the boundaries of their work with each client.

Unfortunately, many of us growing up have been so seriously traumatized that our boundary awareness is flawed. As clients we do not know how to protect ourselves against intrusion. We may invite the abuse we suffered in childhood. As therapists we may ignorantly act out on others our worst injuries, a powerful reminder that the unconscious frequently runs us unaware, that the unconscious really is unconscious.

In recent years teachers, clerics, therapists and doctors have attracted adverse publicity because of the misuse of public trust through inappropriate sexual or other abusive behavior. Bodyworkers, however, do not stand out as miscreants in an otherwise pristine field of ethical esthetes. Because a psychological body therapy utilizes touching, a volatile, powerful technique, a great responsibility attends its use in much the same way as judgement and training are demanded of the police in the use of firearms. There are forms of therapy where any touching is a clear violation of the conventions of the therapeutic form; some therapists cannot conceive of valid touching in an analytic psychotherapy. Our best response to such criticism is to train and monitor our work adequately, so that we do not act out destructively against the client we seek to help, and we assist our clients to develop clear boundaries.

A psychologically-oriented body therapy is remarkably suited to define client boundaries, since body therapy provides physical handles to psychological intangibles. Chapter 12 of this book discusses boundaries and provides exercises to uncover what might otherwise be lost in verbal therapy. Many of the exercises do not include touching by the therapist, as a way of acknowledging the complexity involved with touching. A successful psychologically-oriented bodywork can be conducted, and should be conducted in some cases, without physical contact. As a male therapist working with a woman client, for instance, I may discover in my client's personal history reasons why touch would be misunderstood and provocative. Nevertheless, the client may want to work through these issues with a man rather than a woman. This book cautions against touching until the issues of boundaries and transference/counter-transference have been fully explored.

I must, like all therapists, ride herd on my counter-transference. When I was younger I was too unreflecting and open with my clients. I wanted to "save people" and avoid conflict and hide my separateness. I wanted to heal my mother's inconsolable pain and my father's shame, and I wanted to be acknowledged as a hero. Seasoned over time I still want, too often, to intervene with bright ideas, indulging in a flood of thoughts. My narcissism has scratched its way through the past into the present.

I have become cautious in my use of touch. Partly because I have become humbled by its power, partly because I have become educated to its misuse. Touch is our earliest language, and therefore, capable of taking us back instantaneously to our most primitive universe. It is essential that we always discuss touch with our clients at the beginning of bodywork. Considering carefully the client's history of touch and their expectations for its use, we must touch them never exceeding the emotional level we are working at. We must think carefully about the client's history of touch and their expectations for it's use. We think about their particular dynamics, their character issues, and their current functioning. Diagnosis defines the issues, theory informs our work, but it is the central concern for the client's well being above all else, that delineates how we use touch.

The legal and ethical challenges to our profession have served to educate us about our responsibilities. There is an inherent imbalance in the therapeutic relationship that demands our constant awareness. The client is always the more vulnerable of the dyad, no matter how different the matter might appear outside the therapy chambers. This imbalance is made even more potent in the context of touch. In our culture, people of higher status initiate touch and touch more those of lower status. Men touch women more than women touch men. The imbalance in our society can and does wound. We, as therapists must constantly be aware of the effect our touching is having. We touch, but are not touched. We may be in danger of repeating cultural wounds of gender and class, disempowering rather than awakening. I find that as a man, and as a white male, I must work to stay conscious of my culturally sanctioned "privileges" and invite my clients to question touch in all of its meanings.

How do we differentiate between touch that injures and touch that heals? The sadistic from the empathic, the erotic from the compassionate? As in other theoretical disciplines, we must examine ourselves. Our own therapy and training should be broad and deep, opening as many views to ourselves as possible. We must see our vulnerabilities, grieve our losses, hone our strengths, and come to terms with our limitations. For some of us this is an ongoing and never ending task.

Many of our professional colleagues do not understand the legitimate use of touch in an analytic psychotherapy. They argue that by touching, we merely gratify our own or our clients unconscious desires. By soothing our clients, the unconscious material fails to surface. These are not foolish concerns, even though their absoluteness must be disregarded. The acceptance and meaning of physical contact differs according to the structure, rules and assumptions of the particular therapy. If, as a therapist, I were to adjust my client's head and neck like a chiropractor, massage him like a masseuse, or realign him using techniques of a rolfer, my client would leave bewildered. My touch must be in keeping with the tradition of work and must be judged from the most competent examples of that tradition.

Between the psychoanalytic and the therapeutic world of touch lies and unbridged gulf, a difference in tradition, theory and practice, a difference between a purely intrapsychic and an interpersonal model. Certainly it is undesirable to touch in an intrapsychic drama running five days a week, facilitated by free association, with a mostly invisible therapist, a drama designed to bypass the body. The smallest gesture can feel like an intrusion in the theatre where the lights are turned down on the external world. To a lesser extent in the once a week, face to face psychodynamic psychotherapy, any physical contact take on pregnant meaning, and call for defensive explanation because with the exception of shaking hands, tradition has excluded touch from the psychoanalyst's office.

The taboo of touching was built on an intrapsychic psychology of instinctual repression, a conceptual framework in which touch was believed inevitably to trigger repressed desire and call it forth unsuitably before its time, making the client dependent on the therapist's ego for containment at the expense of his own. This artificial dependence initiated by the therapist serves only the therapist's needs for power and gratification. But working from an interpersonal model as well as an intrapsychic one, we who are psychological body therapists take another viewpoint. The world for us does not dissolve so that all that remains are internal representations and internal conflict. We do not necessarily minimize our presence with every client.

The possibility of problematic responses to touch must not be ignored by somatic therapists. Because of the gulf between the two communities, the psychoanalytic concerns of transference and the misuse of touch have received too little response in somatic literature. Sadly this is because such criticism mostly has been used to dismiss and discredit rather than to encourage dialogue. Within the community of somatic therapy, on the other hand, study and discussions of transference, Object Relations and Self Psychology have been going on for some time.

There are two styles of psychological bodywork. In the first style, talk guiding the client's awareness of her body holds a prominent place. In the second style, talk interferes, pulling the client away from the bodily communication carried out through touch. The pace and timing of each style is different and I suspect the temperament of the therapist preferring each style is different as well; and yet for the somatic therapist it is important to cross over to provide a client with a full range of bodywork. My work has centered around the first style, although I necessarily must step easily into the second style with numbers of clients.

During verbal work, I don't hold my clients nor do I touch them without due cause because a verbal psychotherapy sets a pattern that places touch under scrutiny. Working within this style it feels right to maintain a certain distance in the face of the deep intimacies that are verbally shared. At such times I can feel a desire to physically comfort the client, even though I know I will not do this. I might even imagine contact to be in the best interest of my client. But then I must examine my own behavior. Perhaps my intuition, my kinesthetic self has access to information about myself or my client that I am unaware of. I make a mental note to consult with a colleague who will help me clarify my experience. Then I can return to the crucible of the clinical hour to listen carefully to what is being asked of me.

In style one as therapists we identify character issues and character defenses. We do not rush into bodywork before developing trust with the client and coming to understand the central problems the client faces. We need time to explore the transference relationship. Images bind energy and if we can unearth the underlying image, the character structure lets go with relative ease. Often the body has a truth that it defends through character. Verbally stated, the body might say, "You can't hurt me! I have withdrawn my energy to the core. My legs are tightly muscled and strong. My father beat my legs with a belt." If we work on the withdrawn life in the legs through grounding exercises and kicking, perhaps images of abuse will surface. Unless we get to the underlying image by verbal or bodily means, the body will at some level hold on to the defensive structure. Style one works with the psyche-soma correspondence approaching it from the image or the energy direction. Once the bodywork has begun, a client may need to talk for a session or two to integrate the material triggered by the work. Style one lends itself to building a functional ego, to a psychology of self as well as instincts. Style one addresses the full complexity of the therapeutic encounter.

As well as working with the gift of language, we must work with the gift of silence. Only in silence with the body-standing-up or the body-lying-down can the energetic language of the body be attended to. In style two, words are a distraction. A nonverbal relationship is established which heightens both the body's expression in its many forms and the therapist's attention to body language. In style two, touch becomes the major way in which the therapist responds to a flushing abdomen, deep sighs, tears, spasmodic jerking, deep releases and trembling and the calm waters of easy resting. The therapist's response is often powerful because of its professional quality and its variety: the range of touch: probing, hovering, delicate, comforting, neutral, efficient, cautious, lavish, surrounding, specific, electric, intuitive. Touch can awaken the hidden resources lying fallow in flaccid, undeveloped tissue. Touch can tune each body area to the pulsation of breath, to what Lillemor Johnsen calls the "breathing wave." Some people have wonderful hands. Energy flows through them in an obvious felt rush. Something always happens when they touch. In the language of touch, to not touch may also be eloquent. In style two the practitioner must know when not to interfere because touch can also become a distraction, pulling attention away from the inner process.

Years ago after a particularly moving session with a client lying down, the client returned the next week deeply injured, accusing me of being cold and distant. I was shocked because I had felt close and made supportive and warm statements to her. What mattered to her was that I had not touched her. I might have held her hand. All the rest that I had provided had no meaning to her. I had not responded appropriately to the level she was on, a level that demanded touch. I was functioning from style one while her state of mind called for style two work.

Talk and free association do not always release what is coded at a cellular level. Style two has the advantage of plunging us into the preverbal years when the mother's touch meant everything. We awaken to a body language, unearthing a feeling expression lost to us for years. The glitches in our early expression stand out. This body process breaks the control of the ego, and the defenses so rigidly held begin to shed. All the protections developed with the advent of language hang upon us as dead weight. The head loses its domination and the self locates in chest and belly. The body becomes the unconscious revealing itself and touch the manner of its voice.

Through the client's terror and comfort, the therapist addresses the arrests of a lost time. The therapist takes on the transference of the parent with all the child's destroyed dreams as well as reparative possibilities. The therapy becomes the container that enables the client to grieve his or her early losses and surrender to life as it is now. For the moment only, therapy is comforting. We are not the "good" parents the client needed, and therefore cannot heal him or her of earlier hurts. No, we act as the witness and facilitator to the client's gradual embodiment. Such deep privations require enduring defenses available to the client when we are not. It is then that language mediates and makes bearable the formerly unendurable.

Like fire, touch, is from the gods. It is elemental and essential like dance. Even words "touch" us. There are no alternatives, no replacements. For children touch is food. Not to touch them is abusive. A phobic response to touch strikes against the joy of life. Touch carries the voice of the body. Touch is the vehicle of spiritual healing through the laying on of hands. Touch blesses. Touch, in therapy, for some will seem primitive, unreflective and dangerous, but I believe it is a tool like any other. Any tool can be a weapon. But, used correctly, thoughtfully, judiciously, the tool of touch is a balm that heals ancient wounds long forsaken.

Chapter 3

Counter-Transference

This paper is devoted to the hypothesis that innate among man's most powerful strivings toward his fellow men, beginning in the earliest years and even earliest months of life, is an essentially psychotherapeutic striving. The tiny percentage of human beings who devote their professional careers to the practice of psychoanalysis or psychotherapy are only given explicit expression to a therapeutic devotion which all human beings share.

—Harold F. Searles, *The Patient as Therapist to his Analyst*

We have discussed touch and to some degree transference but there is always more to say about transference. There are many fine books in psychology on transference and I feel no need to duplicate them here. I assume that the reader has a general understanding about transference and its implications in therapy. The issue of counter-transference and body work has been neglected and this chapter attempts a small beginning in the readdressing of that issue. It is by no means meant to be the final word in this crucial area. An opening question could be, how do our bodies inform and enlighten our work with our clients?

Some clients give us energy and others drain us. With experience we can tell that their impact on us is not about our mood. Other clients we see do not effect us in that way. At each meeting, we find ourselves drained or elated. We may be resonating to our client's energy. They may have a similar effect on other people, or we may be experiencing our response because of our own personal history. In either case, this reveals enormously important material about our work with the client. In projective identification a client gets us to feel emotions they have rejected in themselves and thus identify the feelings with us. We may get mad so that our client doesn't have to own his or her own anger. Sometimes certain clients remind us of our critical mother or father and we respond with defensiveness, withdrawal, fatigue and repressed anger. We can study our emotional responses, our visceral responses and write them down in private notes to ourselves. We can attend to any emerging patterns and search out their meanings with a supervisor, therapist or colleague. We then begin to more powerfully use ourselves and our responses.

We are the instrument. By knowing our bodies, we enlarge our understanding and increase our usefulness in the client's therapeutic process. Our vision, however, is also distorted by our uniqueness, our structure, and our vulnerabilities. But by knowing ourselves, including our ragged edges and our depths, we become the fine bone flute we are meant to be. We know our scale and range, we know the best placement of the fingers, we know the sweet pressure of the breath that brings our song to life, and we learn its meaning. By knowing this, we know what is being stirred within us when clients speak. Their voice elicits a tightness in our hearts, we then listen for the echo in our own being, and its meaning in the therapy.

Our bodies are constantly sending and receiving information. In the therapy hour I watch not only the client's energy but also my own. I observe not only the client's breathing and constrictions, but I also attend to my own. At times I might duplicate the client's positioning of arms, legs, head, torso, to gather information from my own body about what such a configuration connotes. I feel what sensations emerge in my own body as the client works. At times images connected to a specific body area will be evoked. For the most part, my own body experiences are background and the client's experience and presentation is foreground. Yet my body is the stream always available, educating me about the client, the therapy, our interaction, and my own being.

Over the years Harold Searles has written a series of articles gathered into a fascinating book on counter-transference. While supervising therapists, he saw that therapy bogged down at the level of the therapist's unexplored unconscious material. Clients then attempt to heal the therapist, who represents a dysfunctional parent. Our bodies and our energetic response provide a direct line to unconscious events in our client as long as we can distinguish our own needs and tendencies. The therapist's unconscious energetic life can impact the client, structuring responses and in some cases interfering with healing.

I worked with a man who seemed to have an energetic wall around him that persuaded me not to touch him. Verbally he invited me to touch but the energy felt thick, dark and impenetrable. I would consider my experiences in this regard as vague and "magical" if I had not had countless energetic impressions confirmed by work with many clients and students. (In fact, I believe this awareness is available to everyone; even the most novice student can perceive energy quite accurately. We all experience each other energetically every day. We see people in a dark mood. We sense that we should or should not approach others. There is nothing mysterious in these daily occurrences because we give them no thought.) It was necessary to talk to my client about the energetic barrier around him to see if he could acknowledge or explain the contradiction he had presented me. As we worked, the client came to realize that he was very conflicted about being close to me, or to anyone. Yet, he felt he "should" let others in. From that point on we began to work with his deepest levels of suffering, retreat, and longing.

When I work with clients I want the unconscious and unspoken made conscious and outspoken, and I want to build mutual understanding. I do not want to collect secret knowledge about a client and not tell information to avoid conflict or hurt feelings. I am not in the client's hire to bear the noble burden of secret knowledge too damaging to share. The clients who experience themselves as too fragile for shared truth tell the therapist in no uncertain terms, and then an agreement can be reached about how to proceed. Usually our attempts to protect our clients are disguised attempts to protect an image of ourselves from client anger and disappointment.

When clients stand, they are being exercised and supported in autonomy. If we are drawn to touch them a lot with no conscious purpose, they may be calling forth the mother and father in us to feed their neediness. We will do well to talk to clients about our pull to comfort them and reflect together about the usefulness of such action. We all work to find a healthy balance between dependence and autonomy. As therapists drawn to help clients, we may seek indirectly to comfort ourselves, unable to bear the pain expressed by their lives. Maybe we wish to save our mother from pain, or secure a more available father, tasks we tirelessly attempt through our clients like Sisyphus pushing his rock. As therapists, we may tremble with awareness, as we allow a new separation to take place, refusing the fantasy that we are merged with our client, who is healed and whole, standing before us.

When a client lies down, another dynamic takes place that calls for discretion and knowledge. Lying down the client is likely to allow certain defensive behaviors to relax, to regress sometimes to a childlike state, to project the good or bad parent onto the therapist, to sexualize the encounter, to enter into a full expression of need, or to split off and become unavailable and "dreamy." The body-lying-down lends itself to touch and to contact in an intimate space. This posture may threaten some therapists and nurture or seduce others. Again, by knowing ourselves, our vulnerabilities, our own patterns of response, we come to know what these responses mean. We come to know what is being called forth from us, its meaning and who calls. The neutrality expected of the therapist is not a deadness but an aliveness that can detach or enter into contact, a reflective and self-possessed presence that intuitively engages and searches out the emotional meaning of the moment.

For some body therapies, the body-lying-down is the only posture provided by the convention of the discipline, and the therapist positions herself to allow maximum body access and movement. In the discipline I practice in which other postures are explored, lying down can be charged with meaning because it represents a choice. Where we position ourselves as therapist is important. If we remain seated in a chair high above the client, our lofty position provides a safe distance or betokens a remote parent. When we sit behind the client's head in a position to touch the face and neck, we are in a position of absolute control. Sitting parallel to the pelvis or opposite the thighs is likely to evoke sexual feelings. Depending on the type of work, therapists move around the body, but the safest place to begin is by one side of the chest close enough to touch or be pushed away and available to be seen. From this starting place the implications of every move can be discussed.

The transference evoked by touch and position are at the heart of a psychological body therapy. Attention to our feelings and countertransference is critical to deep and effective work. Therapists eager to please or prove effective can be drawn to touch clients, hold them, struggle and wrestle with them only to be rejected and hated later. Our willingness to carry out the deep wishes of our clients who are trying to explore repressed memories can lead us to repeat abuse. Sewn in with the wheat of our spontaneous healing impulses are the tares of our darker selves. When clients "open us up" with a moving session, we can not assume that everything that comes from our heart is good therapy. Therapy is never executed on someone else. It is a work we labor at together. When we are doing good work we allow the client as much room and as much access to our skills as possible. The work we do together is in the service of the client. Yet the therapy, like birth labor, is worked through us as well, we, too, are transformed.

Therapy exposes us, the perpetrators of this consuming and dangerous discipline, to ever deepening levels of ourselves, levels of unraveling we never expected. Our commitment must be to come to the truth in ourselves. Because we know this, we know our tatters, we know our tested steel, we can, at our best, be a tool of transformation.

Chapter 4

Seven Tools

We use seven tools in a psychologically oriented body therapy: language, touch, transference, kinesthetic awareness, restructuring, emotional expression, and the psyche-soma correspondence. We have discussed touch and transference. Our use of language deserves no special comment except in its application discussed in the psyche-soma correspondence. I think there is value in listing these tools so that we come to utilize them all in our work with clients. We are likely to be predisposed to a few techniques and ignore other possibilities. Although each is elaborated on in subsequent sections, I present a brief overview here.

Kinesthetic Awareness

Kinesthetic awareness addresses our loss and recovery of bodily feeling, establishing a connectedness that is experienced kinesthetically. A client, when a child, was struck across the face by her alcoholic mother when she was upset. Another client was bent over with the emotional burdens she carried. A third client had no feeling in his legs. They were strong from exercise, but learning to walk had been painful and confusing for him. Apparently his mother could not tolerate his achieving this level of autonomy. In all these cases areas of the body were numb. One client had withdrawn energy and feeling from the left side of her face. Her left eye squinted as if sensitive to the light and she occasionally darted sudden glances in my direction as if I were a threat to her physical safety. The second client had little sensation in her curved, knotted upper back. When I pushed into the tissue on either side of the spine, she hardly felt it. The third client became anxious when he stood with knees bent in a grounding exercise for a few minutes.

Many clients have very little feeling in their bodies. Children learn to manage scary feelings by holding their breath and cutting back the degree of sensation experienced. Withdrawal from parts of our body is a crude but common defense against psychological and physical discomfort. We redirect ourselves through hard and soft exercises, through repeated movements, through light and deep tissue work, to develop kinesthetic awareness. One of the great triumphs in my personal therapy was finally to feel my legs, a modest, yet exquisite, pleasure. Feeling my legs, I was able kinesthetically to sense how they liberated my upper body for movement, providing support and mobility.

Restructuring

Restructuring pertains to our physical and psychological realignment and reintegration. When the client with the bent back discussed the emotional burdens she bore, she blamed others for her trouble. She eventually was able to see how she had created her way of life and maintained her life as burdened. She experienced her ambivalence about straightening up her financial and personal relationships. Her back and her attitude took time to restructure, but she accomplished this with courage and flair.

Emotional Expression

Emotional expression deals with the restrained or cathartic release and the containment of emotional energies. Our *affects* of anger, sadness, pleasure, and joy for example, are momentary responses we hold in common with others of our species, while *emotion* contains our personal history and attitude which transforms, sustains, and amplifies the affect. Our *feeling* has to do with our conscious awareness of emotion and affect. If someone shouts at us briefly, we are startled. If they shout at us in a sustained way, our affect response is anger. How long we hold on to the feeling depends on emotion, on the flood of felt associations that suddenly lean on the present moment. Sometimes growing up we learn to hide our affective response. Perhaps anger is not acceptable in our family. Our emotional life provides the rich color that personal history brings to an affect, qualities that help sustain feeling over time. The good news is that we can hold love in our hearts when the affect isn't being triggered. The bad news is that we can make a mountain out of a molehill. We can hold on to petty resentments and fuel our hatreds with slanderous thoughts.

Often our emotional life is buried in unconsciousness. We do not know how we feel under certain conditions. Facing our boss or lover, everything seems okay, but driving home in the car, we fall into a rage. In a psychological body therapy we explore emotional history to find why present events have particular meaning to our client. Sometimes we discover emotions that are laden with memories that distort the present events and need to be differentiated from them. In a psychologically oriented body therapy, we want our clients to have access to the full range of emotions and have appropriate ways to express emotion. Our emotional history tells us what matters and what the events of our daily lives mean. Without an intimate and immediate connection to our emotional life, our awareness of being present is eroded.

Psyche-Soma Correspondence

In a psychological body therapy we hold the separate forms of body and psyche in our two hands, The body expresses through the interruptions, the withdrawals and the relentless river of energy. Amid halts, unconscious gaps and unearthly stillnesses, the psyche stumbles over itself in the darkness with images caught in momentary flashes of light. With effort a candle of conscious awareness is lit and a sequential world is devised and held together through imaginative leaps across dark spaces. A presumption of self gathers and broods. It is the interplay of psyche's images with energetic flow, most easily identifiable as "character" and revealed through posture, that we call psyche-soma correspondence.

Remarkably, we assume a harmonic flow takes place automatically between these utterly separate realities of psyche and soma. The psyche-soma correspondence as a tool appreciates the separateness as well as the dramatic joining of image and energy. Images bind energy. The image of being beaten emotionally or physically, impressed on us in childhood, can make us cower our whole lives. The image holds us captive until it becomes conscious. Then the body and psyche can liberate its energy. The body often clearly expresses the underlying unconscious image.

Chapter 5

The Four Stages
of Somatic Psychotherapy

> And here you will allow me to somewhat arrogantly and dog-
> matically state that purely medically trained analysts find
> themselves somewhat at a disadvantage, because the whole
> bias of their intellectual training has been to read language
> factually for information, and not as an exercise in imagina-
> tion. Glover's (1968) statement that: 'Fundamentally, the sci-
> ence of psychology is an exercise in imagination,' should
> never be lost sight of in this context.
>
> M. Masud R. Khan, "The Becoming of a Psycho-Analyst"

In conducting a psychological body therapy, it is useful to have a
basic structure in mind. The structure I use encorporates the body-
standing-up and the body-lying-down. The stages are: meeting,
upper body, lower body, and integration. To some degree they cor-
respond to the remaining four sections of this book: contact, character, protest, and embodiment.

Stage One: Meeting

Usually when new clients come in they have a story to tell and a
current problem. Often they arrive in crisis. I write down what they
consider to be the problem, aiming for mutual agreement about
the nature of their problem. I am in danger of drawing conclusions
about clients problems without including their peculiar framework
for their pain. Holding on to their exact words helps me come to

terms with the way they think as distinct from my own process and helps us agree to a therapeutic plan. Some clients, particularly more disturbed clients, need their own language spoken back to them in order to understand what is being said. They don't know me. They do not know what my words mean. Later when giving interpretations, my using the client's language can help the client take in an alien concept. There are six steps to my assessment: presenting problem, history, the black box of childhood, body assessment, mutual understanding and a therapeutic strategy.

In the first session, I explain to my client something of how I work. Each therapist finds a way to describe his or her personal process. I tell them that my process tends to be active. I will share observations with them but that I trust they will know what is true for them and correct me. They must tell me if something I say or do disturbs them. I work to establish a mutual interchange where understanding can be "hashed out." There are times in therapy when I am a silent witness to clients' stories. It is more useful for them to have the safe environment to explore their thoughts and feelings uninterrupted. Ideally as therapists we have the flexibility to shape ourselves appropriately to the clients' therapeutic need.

In the first few sessions I explore the presenting problem and take down a personal history and a medical history. If sexual problems are mentioned as one of the presenting complaints, I take a sexual history. I do not start bodywork during a crisis. Even the most benign exercises in bodywork can open psychic doors with clients. I like to take time to build some basic understandings with my client before I actually do bodywork with them.

The progression of the exercises set down in this book is designed to begin with the least threat to clients and the most opportunity to gather further knowledge about the client. These early exercises assist the client in developing awareness about themselves. If we employ techniques that "open up" the client disregarding their fear and their boundaries, we can stumble into buried rage, terror and memories that cause the client to retreat from further deep work for months.

When all the history has been taken there usually remains the black box of early childhood. We can see what came out of the black box but we cannot see inside. What we cannot see, we imagine. Much of psychology hypothesizes about the possibilities that take place during that time when developing patterns determine personality structure unconsciously for the rest of our lives. Psychology creates a healing myth specific to our culture and supported by our developing knowledge of childhood. With the client we build a picture of the past and its style of intrusion in the present. Through our theories we frame our clients problems in a form that invites resolution.

At this time in the history of psychology, children and childhood relationships are being extensively studied by practitioners and researchers. We know something about a child's developmental stages, however, our clients often cannot remember very much of their early childhood. Clients often remember parents at the beginning of therapy as better or worse than they do at the conclusion of our work. Although the early development of the child's sense of having a separate self is not something the client remembers, we can see from the problems and behaviors of our client that this early period supported or did not support self development. Our work needs to address those early injuries, to define them and seek ways to build a functional and durable self. The study of the false self (character), addressed in the third section, reveals the limited options possible to a child building defenses.

The first task of an analytic psychotherapy is to help a client identify the false self that he or she has developed to accommodate as a child to the perceived parental demands. This mask of accommodation as defensive structure compensates for failures in development. The false self blocks healing. It hides a weakness and prevents our core nature from dealing with fear, pain, anger, excitement, desire and loss. My task is to identify the defensive character and help the client differentiate her/himself from her/his parents. But to this noble plan some clients may not have the slightest interest. Seemingly abstract explanations mean nothing to them. We must work concretely with the problem in the present, approaching the past that's in the black box and perhaps never getting inside.

When clients come in for body psychotherapy, I ask them to

stand at a distance from me of at least six feet and to close their eyes and notice what they feel in their bodies. I watch their movements for several minutes. I look at the posture, the holding, the body slumps, collapses, rigidities, and I look for the strengths and innate resources that the body presents. (It is difficult to describe what I look for so as to be fully understood. This entire book is training for this moment of observation. "The Individual Signature of the Body" in this section will guide you through the initial body process.) For further evaluation I use the eight stations, described in Section Three, as a measure for restructuring. And I use the time to reflect on an appropriate therapeutic strategy. After a few minutes I ask the client what he or she has noticed and I reflect back to him/her some impressions of the structural patterns.

When I look at the body structure, I am looking for a therapeutic strategy that includes what I know of my client's personal history. After having discussed with the client his/her presenting problems and also reflected about the personal history, I usually explore defensive strategies that may impinge on the client's present life. I seek supportive evidence from early memories of childhood as well as current family patterns. Character provides the crossover from psyche to body. Alexander Lowen, a student of Wilhelm Reich, defined five character structures (see chapter 15) which relate to the developmental stages of childhood and have a psyche-soma correspondence. With many clients I come to a mutual understanding of the particular and the more general problems facing them. We agree on a therapeutic plan.

Some clients do not see me initially for body psychotherapy. After we work together for a while and the immediate crisis resolves, I may suggest a body psychotherapy as the most useful direction. For instance, a person who is extremely verbal with little access to emotion or a person who feels dissociated from body experience might profit from the gradual introduction of bodywork. For some clients a study of the false self and relationships with family members on a verbal level is the preferable way to proceed. After a longer period of therapy, I'll suggest bodywork, a study of dreams, or a combination of dreams and the body. Even when the psychological structures of defense have been understood and adjusted psychologically, the body often continues to hold the old patterns knowing no way to let go of old rigidities. Bodywork helps the client release the rigid holding that psychologically he or she has now outgrown.

Stage Two: Upper Body

After the explorations of Stage One, in Stage Two we bear down, primarily, to break through chronic holding in the upper body. In order for the upper body to "let go," the support of the lower body needs to be felt, and so we also work on the legs with the body-standing-up to establish a deep ground. Whereas in Stage One we were content with insight and tentative exploration, in Stage Two we have decided on a course of actions. We work with the ocular, oral and cervical segments to clear blocks to the energy flow, and then we work to free up the holding in the chest. In Stage Two we have the cooperation of the client and sufficient knowledge of the bodily condition to press hard to restructure.

During a grounding exercise (standing with knees bending with the rhythm of breathing) in Stage One we would have allowed a client to stop the exercise when faced with discomfort. In Stage Two we encourage the client to allow the vibration to intensify and endure the pain of chronically held muscle. The work of Stage Two often calls for patience and focused attention in order to restructure successfully. When the character armor is confronted forcefully, the client may feel anxiety. Frequently, memories and intense feeling emerge after the therapy session. Clients need to be warned to be observant and sometimes careful during the week. We don't want our clients falling into therapy-related unbounded rages at inopportune times, while driving the car for instance.

Stage Three: Lower Body

In Stage Three we bring the upper and lower body together. Feeling in the pelvis opens up and energy begins to flow. For the many people who have blocked all feeling connection to the pelvis, any feeling will be experienced as sexual or painful. Often people are frightened by pelvic sensation. The techniques of Stage Three tend to be softer, allowing a melting of armor rather than a breaking through. Many exercises of this stage are carried out lying down, although streaming (unblocked energetic flow) can take place standing up also. The orgasm reflex may establish itself at this stage. With the completion of Stage Three we can expect a better connection between the head, the heart and the genitals. In Stage Three and Four we bring the warmth and contact of our hands to the hypotonic musculature, those underdeveloped body areas. We call forth the repressed memories and the resources of the body-lying-down.

Stage Four: Integration

In Stage Four we consider the body as a whole and we restructure and integrate splits. We revisit old exercises and body themes where we found deficits. We work with movement, dreams and bodily expression. We are freer to take the somatic work into spontaneously motivated directions. The domination of the basic character structure has been broken. Transference issues come to resolution, allowing the client to be more aware of the therapist's limitations and to separate from the the therapist. The therapist must tolerate the loss of the client's dependent posture toward her. Some clients do not reach this stage. It is enough to have joined head, heart and genitals and have exercises available to sustain the gains they have made.

Even with these aids to a psychologically based bodywork, the beginning therapist will stumble in confusion. We are not body-oriented in life or therapy and it takes years to incorporate bodywork into our practice. With time the work becomes elegant and powerful and sometimes miraculous. Even with a verbal psychotherapy we come to make many somatic observations which support the analysis.

Chapter 6

Equipment

This chapter deals with useful equipment: the barrel, the stool, the basketball, the plastic bat, the rolled blanket, the cube, small balls, the broom handle or dowel, and the towel. It is my preference to work without special equipment. Simplicity is elegant, but at times useful function takes priority.

The Stool

The stool is modeled after the padded arm of a sofa and can be made from a stool roughly 23 inches high with a rectangular seat. Upon this a tightly rolled army blanket is strapped down with bungie cords. When our back is stiff and rigid, standing we can lean backward onto the stool taking care not to tip it over. The stool is confrontive and effective. The ideal position for it is mid-back at the diaphragm, although it is important to use the stool to loosen the upper and lower back too. The task is to let go and relax, and let the pelvis sink down. The first few rides on the stool should be brief to get acquainted with its surprising virtues. The therapist should guide the client getting off the stool, which may tip over unless the client crouches down. After using the stool it is useful to do a bend-over (exercise 12), to bend the other way.

The Barrel

The barrel, 18 inches in diameter, is usually constructed from a heavy cardboard tube core wrapped in foam and covered in a fabric. Sitting on the floor leaning against the barrel, the client finds it easy and safe to roll his/her back against the solid, comforting form. I allow clients to explore the barrel's possibilities before I ask them to assume a particular position. Like the stool, the barrel's central position is opposite the diaphragm at the midback. I like to start clients with their necks against the barrel so that slowly as they roll, they can feel the pull of the neck muscles anchored to the upper back.

The Basketball and Rolled Blanket

A basketball is particularly helpful for clients to use at home. A basketball is easily available. The ball can be pumped up soft or hard, and provides a more specific pressure, but less stability than the barrel. The basketball is excellent for releasing the lower back and sacral area. When clients lie over it face up, their shoulders ground on the floor. A tightly rolled blanket on the floor is another way available to clients to open up the back and chest. The client, lying on the floor, positions the rolled blanket between the back and the floor to stretch the back and chest.

Small Balls and Dowels

A baseball, tennis ball or rubber ball are great to roll under the feet. Our feet with so many bones and muscles have been stuck in shoes and molded to a seemingly solid mass. The balls loosen up the feet and restore them to life and feeling. A more painful but effective way to awaken the feet is to go over a broom handle or dowel laid on the floor or rug, an inch at a time. A baseball can be useful for clients in other areas of the body. One of my clients recently suffered from painfully contracted muscles in his hip and lower back. He was delighted to find relief by lying on the floor and gently pressing the tender area against the baseball. The muscles relaxed.

The Cube and Towel

I use a 24 inch square foam cube in four ways. Clients often hit the cube with a plastic toy bat or with their fists and forearms. They may lie over the cube on their bellies keeping their balance with their feet while I work on their backs. Clients can kick the cube if I brace it with my legs. Holding the cube up, I invite clients to wear garden gloves and punch the cube. The cube provides protection and proximity. When a client hits or kicks the cube I hold, there is an interchange. Is his anger unleashed at me? I can feel the energy and read the expression and inquire. Sometimes instead of hitting, a quality of rage can best be expressed by twisting a towel, like wringing a person's neck. Twisting a towel will call up submerged anger in some clients.

Chapter 7

Staring, Clothing,
and the Inequities of Power

Some years ago in an internship, I worked in Juvenile Hall talking
to and testing adolescents and writing court reports requested by
probation officers. I was at ease with adolescents, having taught
English for years before I trained in psychology. So I was taken
aback when my first young client confronted me in a hostile tone,
"What are you staring at?" Children know that staring is a power
strategy. Parents can see when a child is lying. Children avert their
eyes or brazenly stare back before the severe questioning eyes of
authority. As a teacher I had never been aware of how I used my
eyes. They were not a threat in a private school classroom of middle class tenth graders. But to a youth in trouble, my stare was
frightening and insulting. He taught me a great deal. I was no help
to him at all.

I discovered that I relied on sight to pick up all my cues about
people. I studied their faces and bodily shifts as if my intuitions
were restricted to this one sense alone. But after my first serious
failure I consciously averted my eyes with kids. I let them study
me. I allowed them the dominance and let them come to know
me. Rather than stare and pry verbally, I looked elsewhere and
talked generally. Invariably, they came to the point themselves.
They interrupted my prattle with direct statements like, "My
mother's boyfriend is drunk all the time."

I draw a distinction between staring and looking. When we
look, our gaze is relaxed, moving in response to the object of our

attention. We are grounded and present. When we stare, we gaze fixedly, without apparent feeling. Many adults in therapy don't seem to object to being stared at. Perhaps they accept it as the necessary price of therapy or are inwardly preoccupied and don't notice. There are times when I unthinkingly stare at clients, but I have learned to vary my visual routine for this reason. I want to open up all my senses to learn from my clients. I want to break my unconscious fixation on staring and shift my attention to hearing the voice and sensing the body's energy kinesthetically. I think of the whole body as a radar screen. I don't even have to look at the client to know what is going on. In a bodywork session to break away from staring is a liberation and an awakening.

In training groups I have consistently been told by beginners that at first they feel awkward looking at someone's body, and at the same time they feel relieved to have permission to do so. In our culture we tacitly agree not to stare at each other. Staring is intrusive. Staring reduces people to objects. Staring is a visual monologue, not a dialogue; it avoids relationship. Staring represents a lack of contact by overriding the social gestures of the other. Staring overrides boundaries. At other times, we may stare without seeing, looking within. Our clients have hired us to look gently at them rather than stare, to engage them from our grounded selves where we are able to join empathically and return to a separate self.

When we give ourselves permission to look rather than stare at another person, to scan them and note how they move, we break a taboo which has cut us off from each other and ourselves. In workshops we begin with participants acting as client and therapist, standing facing each other. Both the therapist and the client feel exposed. Who has dominance? Are they looking or staring at each other? They laugh and distract themselves to dissolve their social embarrassment and defuse any aggressive aspects of looking at each other as separate and different rather than similar and joined.

When I work with a client in front of groups, I am often overwhelmed with my own body constriction. Now with eyes fixed on me, my shoulders rise in fear. Am I being stared at? Until this moment, when I have been called on to work with someone else, I have been deeply asleep in sensing my body. It's as if I have stepped out of bed after a hard night. Perhaps I am afraid of my own aggression and have projected it onto others. Tradition has us work without shoes to better ground ourselves, but I cannot feel the ground. I adopt a nonchalance to hide my discomfort. I work first with myself. I stretch. I comment on my own tightness, bring myself into kinesthetic awareness, and awaken to my own needs for ground and inner presence. I am not "working on" someone while I stare in safe detachment. There is a powerful energetic exchange in relating as a vulnerable human being. Now I am ready to greet the client. After we have "met" each other, I suggest that the client close his or her eyes for a minute and just notice what he or she feels inside.

In my private practice I begin much the same way. There are, of course, no external observers, but I must also call myself back to myself. I recover the ground that brings me home, to the body where I begin. In these initial sessions, I watch the client's body shift and change in silent ease. With the eyes closed, the client can turn her attention to an internal world. I want to see how acquainted she is with the inside and how she reports her experience. Does her mind run on obsessively seeking protection and escape? Does she have any kinesthetic awareness? Often when the verbal and environmental distractions are removed, the client reports body shifts and sensations that reveal a developing kinesthetic awareness. It is important for the therapist to support the client's kinesthetic awareness by listening attentively rather than parading special knowledge.

Closing ones eyes when someone is close is threatening to many people. Generally clients like lots of space around them. So it is advisable to begin work at a safe distance of eight or ten feet. The therapist moves closer only as the work progresses, and after she checks boundaries and the client's feelings at each step. Nor does the therapist go entirely by what the client says. She watches the body's responses and discusses any discrepancies. Many people have covered their history of abuse with a social pretense of ease. In an initial session the therapist focuses on the basics of contact and studies the eyes for fear, blankness, engagement, humor, aliveness, coldness or the invisible inner barrier that forms the only boundary a person may be able to sustain. "You can do what you want," they seem to say, "but you won't reach my heart."

I believe in watching a client for a long time. I watch the shifts as the minutes pass. I want to "understand" before I "do." The body posture that initially stands before us is not the same as the body posture standing before us five minutes later. Where to begin? What unconscious movements has one observed? Are they relevant? Is it appropriate to move closer at all? Many beginning therapists look only for a place to begin and then stop looking. But what is the overall structure in the body? Are the legs cut off from energy? Are the knees locked, the ankles collapsed, the pelvis rigidly forward? Or the chest collapsed, the head and neck thrust forward in compensation, the chin tilted upward and to the side to cut off from the body? Are the shoulders frozen up and forced back? There are so many ways to begin, so much to observe. Some young therapists become rooted to one spot. They fail to move around from side to side. They stare rather than "take in" the client's presence.

One must look at tissue as well as structure, the energy of the tissue, how it gathers itself, the reluctance of its undeveloped nature or its overbounded character. At a much younger age our bodies shifted to accommodate and settled into compromises and unresolved somatic ambivalences that established themselves structurally. The tissue is dynamic in one place and unearthly still and cold in another.

In long term work a moment by moment reactive approach is deadly. Beginning therapists want to grab onto something fast or they may mindlessly introduce an exercise that addresses a basic issue like grounding or boundaries, harmless in a way but often just as meaningless. Long term goals and a clear plan addressing character armor are essential for structural change. And so our study of the client must explore the psychologically based body structure to design a workable model for change. Lowen's characters are useful in formulating a strategy, but our energy reading of the client will provide the initial steps in unraveling complex defenses.

When I was trained in Bioenergetics we took off clothes and wore only underwear, a bathing suit or shorts and a tee shirt. I threw out my old underwear and bought bright colors. At first we were anxious and uncomfortable being almost naked in front of others. Nevertheless, as a learning experience, it was important to see the flesh pale with energetic withdrawal or flush with engagement. There is excitement in knowing what lies beneath the modesty of clothes. To be fixed on erotic body parts is to miss the point entirely. The whole body is everything William Blake said and drew, a transformative, awakening angel for the moment touching down.

As psychotherapists we brace ourselves against the power of bodily life. We cover private parts as if that protects us from God's gaze. We put on the glasses of science and assume the dignity of one who touches a specimen, exercising a professional distance. We are not meant to gawk at the fiery angel that might turn and destroy us. Even the body's pain and deadness is too alive for us. We can barely tolerate the body's oil and smell. Our body armor becomes our protector against the vibrancy of the body before us. Intellectually we select out what is useful for our therapeutic engagement. We, too, are good at restricted contact.

I have found it unnecessary for clients to disrobe. The fiery angel shines through. Also I push clients to report their own perceptions rather than depending on the all knowing professional, Dr. Know-it-all, to inform them about their own bodies. Bodywork is an easy situation for the professional to assume airs of magical powers. "You utterly amazing person, how did you know that!" It is far better to use our observing powers to confirm or direct our clients' observations, supporting them to develop kinesthetic awareness. Sometimes, of course, there are areas that need to be touched to be known. The hands have powerful eyes to search out the dark energies. Sometimes clients wear loose clothing which covers them but allows momentary exposure of an area.

In the 1960s and early 1970s, everyone mindlessly threw off their clothes on any occasion, but now we have entered a more thoughtful period. It makes sense to respond to the demands of the time without making clothes/no clothes right or wrong. The disrobing of the client, while understandably useful, introduces transference issues that need to be addressed.

What does it mean that we as therapists, fully clothed, look at a client in underwear? Underwear throws us into intimate space. It is what we wear in and out of the bathroom before going to bed. Underwear is for our lover and our family. Underwear can also be for the doctor's examination room. Is association with the doctor what protects our client from exposure? Am I, the therapist, an intimate or an examining doctor?

Societal assumptions about loose shirts and shorts are more neutral and therefore, these clothes are preferable. But what about the inequality of dress? What would it suggest for the therapist to appear in shorts and a shirt also? Tradition supports the inequality of dress, and in individual therapy the therapist's dressing down would be a violation. These transference issues have been discussed for years among body therapists and in training programs.

The truth is that there is a difference between us. The therapeutic relationship has built-in inequities. These inequities are its primary vulnerability and strength. It is the engine that drives the transference. We can use this imbalance consciously to explore and reveal relational issues, or we can ignore it to our great peril. The difference in dress, with all its implications, represents only one layer of transference issues we need to consider in the therapy session. Like the issue of touch, the meaning of physical exposure must be discussed by the therapist and client.

The therapist is under an obligation to examine his own motivation around preferences for client's dress in the bodywork session. In a good training program, therapists learn to hold themselves accountable to their peers. Deviation from the training model in this area, needs to be held suspect. We are not lone wolves, brilliant clinicians operating among docile followers. However dazzling our personal gifts, we remain flawed, ordinary human beings, susceptible to our own vulnerabilities, shadowiness and ignorance. We need peers to help us stay related, in contact, autonomous but interdependent. In recovery from our own worlds of suffering, we too place ourselves in our proper place, as wounded healers.

Chapter 8

The Individual Signature of the Body

There is for each of us a characteristic posture, a body signature, which identifies us. The individual signature distinguishes itself from "character" by representing not only our armoring, but also an aspect of our core nature. We observe a person eating, his head tilted to the right and eyes rolling to the left as he laughs. Even without focusing on facial detail, across a restaurant we know who that is. The way a person sits in a chair or walks on the street may amuse us in its individual style. We may identify friends at a great distance from the lyrical movement of their walk. We catch their spirits in their identifying signatures. Our individual signature is affected also by our family surroundings. Alfred Adler noted that the tree on the top of the mountain looks different from the tree at the bottom. An eldest child will be organized differently than the youngest.

Three Signatures

When we ask a client to stand, we can observe three signatures: an initial signature, a shadow signature and a core signature. During the first few minutes, the posture may be self-conscious, awkward, jumbled or unnaturally still. We are seeing how clients initially gather and present themselves, which is useful information for understanding our client. Sometimes we see a somatic mask hastily put on and other times we see our client's painful vulnerability.

After the first few minutes, the posture resolves to a settled pre-disposition. This second signature, the shadow signature, represents our character, our postural attitude. One shoulder may be higher, the pelvis locked forward or back, the weight predominantly on one leg or other, the chin up or head craned forward. If the spine is unsteady, the discomfort of standing discloses a strained ambivalence. Sometimes the shadow signature is obscured by a forced "correctness," a posture the person learned from the army, karate, or dance.

The shadow signature shows the body compromised without recourse—the body in the midst of war, blood dried in the wound, uncomfortable, rigid and cold, bandaged roughly and covered up. In spite of the shadow, the core signature may be seen through a certain turn of the head, a look in the eye, a certain body style that endures as a natural energetic disposition, a individual expression of humanity. We are so much more than our defenses. When we relax, our being may spontaneously demonstrate themselves through posture and gesture.

In body therapy we seek to support the body in its natural function and core signature. We do not support "correct" movement. Everything living has a twist to it. Something is always a little out of sync, a something unique to our spontaneous expression. Some Japanese potters have wheels which are off-center and they create exquisite beauty without rigid symmetry. So, we are working to interrupt body rigidities that bend us over and twist us into immobility. We are realigning ourselves to create increased flexibility rather than to fit into a superimposed model of straight and tall. Our essential nature does not need fixing. Our beauty is not a possession but the life that flows through us.

Some people, when they walk into a room, turn every head. What is beauty if not, first of all, a miraculous energy? Some people are a blessing on the planet who by just walking around, serve better than wise words or reason. Their being is a profound gift which radiates to others. The youth are often given energy in such abundance that they overrun all their dark holes of withdrawal and despair through the biological pumping of what seems like endless resources. Nothing shuts them down for long. I call it "biological optimism." If you are depressed, it is good to hang out around youth. The abundance of nature, its profusion and generosity, is a gracious gift. Energy overrides even the dark lines of age. To observe energy, we must be able to look longer than a minute. When we take the time, we can observe in others how their initial stance settles into their shadow signature. We may see, too, the core signature and find ways to support that energetic structure.

EXERCISE ONE: STANDING MEDITATION

> There is an essential difference between consciousness and awareness, although the borders are not clear in our use of language. I can walk up the stairs of my house, fully conscious of what I am doing, and yet not know how many steps I have climbed. In order to know how many there are I must climb them a second time, pay attention, listen to myself, and count them. Awareness is consciousness together with a realization of what is happening within it or of what is going on within ourselves while we are conscious.
>
> Moshe Feldenkrais, *Awareness Through Movement*

Someone once instructed me that the mind in meditation is similar to a pool stirred by wind. Thoughts and activity trouble the surface of the mind so that we can not see deeply within. When the wind stills, the pool clears to its deepest place. The movement of our thought in free association leads us inevitably into depths in a manner puzzling to our linear minds. In this meditation we become observers of our thoughts, feelings, and images as they come upon us. For a moment we are swept up in a concern, but we return to a posture of quiet observation. Attention to the thoughts, rather than opposition to them, helps us clear ourselves and return once more, possibly to another level of inner experience. Gradually we come into greater balance, more grounded in a deeper being, less identified with intellect or feeling.

In a standing meditation we observe our thoughts as well as our body of energy. Just as we observed the mind's free association, so we extend to observe the body's free association through movement. In standing, our body shifts as it meets and sloughs off bodily attitudes and ambivalences. The act of standing is complex and touches into the gains and disappointments of early childhood. Standing touches into early unresolved emotional and physical injuries. To feel our emotional, physical awkwardness and ambivalence in therapy relates us to ourselves at the deepest levels.

As I mentioned earlier, when I begin a body therapy session, I often have the client stand with eyes closed for a few minutes to build their awareness. The standing meditation is an attitude toward ourselves that furthers our embodiment. Ask your client to stand at a 6 foot distance from you. Ask her to close her eyes for a few minutes, and notice any feelings she experiences in her body. After a few minutes, ask her what she noticed.

As therapist observers, we find ourselves assessing a number of inadvertent movements that may or may not hold significance. Observe the small movements, shifts in the stance, unconscious movements like twitches, facial expressions and many other details of a body-standing-up. You are forming a general impression of the emotional quality of the posture. "He looks depressed." "She looks burdened." "He looks above it all." Seek out specific body characteristics that support your impressions. Notice areas of the body that seem more alive and areas that impress you as lifeless. While you are paying attention, so is the client. You will probably be pleasantly surprised at how much your observations and impressions are validated by your client's report of his or her inner experience.

Unconscious Movement

In time our attention will be drawn to the body's unconscious movement. Every day, we make hundreds of movements which are perfectly understandable to ourselves and others as necessary actions. We open and close doors, stand up, and stretch. If we observe any of these actions carefully, we notice an individual signature rich in unconscious influences. When a person sits down, he may lower himself down in a controlled, gradual way. Another person might suddenly drop into the chair. Why does one person slide unnoticed through a doorway with eyes averted and another fill the doorway with presence and challenge? Automatic, functional movements reveal our individual signature.

People make unexpected body gestures which appear unrelated to any intended action. A man twitches by lifting his left shoulder suddenly an eighth of an inch. He does not notice the movement himself. He scratches his leg periodically. His foot jerks, he sighs, he squints, his stomach rumbles. These movements are part of the body's voice telling its story without benefit of consciousness. If I am working with a client, I scan her body for unconscious movement. Often I note five or more unconscious movements and then must decide which of these is worth bringing to awareness. Some of these movements, when explored, have emotional significance and meaning. A client taps her foot. "I'm restless ... well actually I'm nervous. I'm always nervous. I don't want to be here. I'm feeling mad." I ask another client "What does that tiny shrug mean with your left shoulder?" She tells me that she used to shrug as a teenager when her mother complained about her brother.

EXERCISE TWO: UNCONSCIOUS MOVEMENT

Ask your client to stand for five minutes while you observe any unexpected, inexplicable movements. Choose two movements which you sense have significance and ask the client to repeat those gestures. Then ask the client what images and feelings arise.

EXERCISE THREE: OBSERVING INDIVIDUAL SIGNATURE

While your client stands with eyes closed taking account of her physical and emotional feelings in a standing meditation, watch her move from the initial to the shadow signature. Take notes or hold the specific body shifts in memory being attentive to their exact order.

We have forgotten the trials and pain involved in the difficult task of standing. Watch how the body shifts over time. Notice the ambivalence in the stance itself, how the upper body shifts, how the spine seems to have trouble holding to one position. Do the

49

shoulders ride up high? One higher than the other? Is the line of the pelvis higher on one side? Draw a stick figure and include lines indicating the slant of the shoulder and pelvis. Notice the tilt of your client's head. Does one shoulder twist forward? Does the hip on the same side rotate forward or reverse the twist? Indicate if the feet point in or outward.

What is your overall impression of the body? What animal does this person remind you of? Do any phrases come to mind? One of my clients looked like a tree clinging to the side of a mountain, another like a bear. Another looked like a bereft six-year-old, the tears dried on her cheeks.

Now stand to the side to see the person's profile. Draw a line indicating the contour of the head, neck and back. Does the head crane forward? Is the chest collapsed or puffed up? What is the slope of the pelvis: riding forward, tucked under or arched back? Does your client lock her knees? If you view from the back, does it look like the back and front belong to different bodies? Let your drawing indicate many of these observations.

A man in his forties whom I've been working with for a few months stands before me. He has stood in a standing meditation at least fifteen times before. When he first stands, his initial signature is evident. His bear-like body is out of touch with itself. His right shoulder is awkwardly raised and twisted back and his knees are locked. The weight of his body appears to press him down. Gradually, as he comes into himself, he makes adjustments. He feels his shoulder and brings it forward. The knees unlock and he brings his chin down.

He is making corrections, but his shadow signature is relatively uneffected. He cannot throw off the bunched and frozen muscle around his neck and shoulders that pulls the back of his head down and thrusts his chin up and forward. The subtle collapse of his mid-chest that restricts his breathing is covered by bulky muscle. Even though he has bent his knees, he does not feel how rigidly he holds his pelvis or know how dissociated he is from his legs. The shadow signature is where our work begins. Through kinesthetic awareness he may develop flexibility and create postural alternatives.

When I see him standing there, I like him. He is an extremely bright and kind man. Qualities of humor and self reflection flash in his eyes. In spite of its rigidity, his body has vitality. He is a man who hugs his children and is unafraid of touch. Something in his posture shows his readiness to engage. I am looking at his core signature, a powerful energetic reality.

EXERCISE FOUR: BODY SCULPTURE

Observe your client for five minutes standing. To intensify kinesthetic awareness, exaggerate and then reverse distinctive postural features. If one shoulder is higher and pushed forward, exaggerate the movement slightly and ask your client how the position feels as he holds the sculpted form. Reverse the posture i.e., lower and push back the shoulder, and ask how that feels. The process of exaggeration and reversal provokes a somatic re-evaluation of balance, moving towards a more moderate posture. The deeper and more lasting purpose, however, remains the increase of kinesthetic awareness, the foundation for somatic change.

Observing the three signatures is a form of life drawing, a central discipline we return to repeatedly. We roughly sketch the shifting pose and capture the body's pose in our mind's eye. What we labored over years before may now become noticeable in a glance. There is, after all, no great variety to the shadow signature. I was informed once that there are only nine basic story plots in the world. All stories can be found to be derivative expressions of these basic forms. There may as well be only nine basic characters and nine basic postures and nine basic attitudes. I would not argue if someone said there were eight or ten instead. Our personalities are limited. Our collapsed chest and our burdened back do not define us as special. But our deep nature, the life that moves us, dreams us and speaks us, does not reduce to stereotypes. We may catch some element of our being in the core signature.

Section Two

Contact and Kinesthetic Awareness

Chapter 9

Contact

The greatest magician among the psychoanalysts and without doubt the most important human personality of them all was Georg Groddeck. I met him in Sweden in 1924 and was immediately fascinated by his veritably diabolical face that looked at me as if from a fiery furnace of hell and yet was so full of deep goodness. My heart went out to him in an almost maternal way, for I felt the enormous vulnerability of his soul which protected itself by spikiness and play-acting.... It is difficult to describe in detail what it was that made Groddeck's Wei Wu so magical. On the whole it probably was his own completely relaxed naturalness.

Hermann Graf Keyserling, Spectrum of Europe

All of us have experienced states of distraction. At such times we forget where we put our keys. Today we are in a hurry; tomorrow we are depressed. Our breathing is shallow and we are not sure how we feel about anything. To be fully present represents a significant achievement barely within the realm of possibility. Beyond the basic principles of contact offered in the following pages, our individual presence builds force through the difficulties we have faced, endured and mastered. Our presence develops from our self acceptance and ruthless honesty with ourselves. We gather our full nature to us in all its darkness and light and embody it as Georg Groddeck did. This book is about being embodied and present here and now.

As children, according to Wilhelm Reich, we were emotionally present until through repressive behaviors of our caretakers and the culture, we turned back upon ourselves establishing a false self, called "character." In part, withdrawn from our true nature, we still found it necessary to fabricate contact. Elusiveness has a certain charm for a while, but failures in contact bring us crippled relationships and emotional futility.

Making contact is more than talking to someone, more than looking at them or touching them. To be in contact, we need to be grounded, have adequate boundaries, enjoy unrestricted breathing, have access to feeling and have the intention to be present. To be fully present reflects a functional and durable sense of self. When someone talks with us, trades looks, and touches us and is not present with us, the experience can feel eerie. Someone who is demonstrative and overflows with feeling may not be in contact. Imagine growing up with parents who never made true contact with you. How then can you be in contact with yourself? Some of us were emotionally pushed and pulled by parents and teachers. In the face of manipulation, we learned to hide while appearing to respond. If a parent never wanted to know who we were, generated all manner of assumptions about us, intruded upon us and never sought our deep agreement in relationship, we may avoid real contact with others automatically, defensively. However, we cannot blame our upbringing for every failure to be present. Genetically we may be predisposed to withdraw from others. We may suffer from shyness and a painful introversion.

In the movie *The Wizard of Oz*, Dorothy, the tin man, the straw man and the cowardly lion cower before the immense, stern image of the wizard. Dorothy's little dog sniffs out behind a curtain the real wizard manipulating a powerful, projected image through dials and levers. In truth, he is a small, insecure, blustering old man. At that moment, real contact is made, not so ideal or magical, but the foundation for real change. We intuit the real. Like a dog, we sniff out the truth. The best liars have to fool the dog, intuition, and that's hard.

Margaret Mahler, in her studies of mother-child relationships, observed difficulties that mothers and babies underwent as they learned to separate from each other for short periods through either crawling or walking. Some children were afraid to step away from the mother and some mothers were fearful to allow their children to leave. A child needs parental support to separate from the parents. In *The Drama of the Gifted Child,* Alice Miller discusses how critical it is that children be acknowledged as important and separate from their parents, that they must be adequately "mirrored". If the child is treated as a mere extension of the parents needs and life attitudes, the child is unlikely to grow up with a solid sense of self apart from others.

Since relationship is fundamentally built on the capacity to appreciate someone who is other than ourselves, unexplored early psychological injury makes genuine relationship difficult. Having suffered early childhood injury, we may seek constant approval or deny that we care at all. We imitate life with a false self. We grow up ungrounded in ourselves, without clear or flexible boundaries. Our breathing is inhibited, but we assume we are present and live without awareness of how distant we are.

Reich experienced a wall of contactlessness with some clients. The lack of contact, he said, resulted from a concentration of ambivalent opposing responses. One passive dependent patient, after some therapeutic work, still appeared to be indifferent to the world. Reich understood this client's underlying indifference to have originated during childhood. When the patient was small, his mother had encouraged closeness and awakened sexual feeling while rejecting the child's advances. As a result, the child, and later the man, harbored a rage toward women while being irresistibly drawn to them. This disturbing conflict was quieted by repressing his rage which resulted in severe loss of feeling. He failed in genuine contact and compensated for it with a seeming contact, a substitute contact.

When we experience contact with someone, we see simplicity and natural expression. We see the range of affect with nothing left out. We see sadness, fear, love, anger, joy, and peacefulness. With substitute contact, something rigid reduces the subtle interplay of feeling to one or two modes of expression. Some people are overly friendly, inappropriately polite, or reserved to a fault. They may be laughing abrasively, assuming intimacy prematurely, acting seductive independent of a particular audience, or oozing charm from every pore. Others dominate conversations without allowing response, and still others act helpless and needy. When we see these behaviors, we may be witness to a substitute contact, an avoidance of deep feeling.

EXERCISE FIVE: INTENTION

In this exercise, we become aware of how we avoid, or make contact. At a distance of an arms length or more, look into your client's eyes to determine how present the client is. The client is encouraged to look into your eyes to determine whether you seem to be present. It has been said that the eyes are the windows of the soul, but they are often boarded up. You may, for instance, look into someone's eyes and see nothing while they look guilelessly unthreatening. Some people always win at staring contests. We may not intend to be present. We may "tune out" while appearing to listen. Another person's eyes may be open to receive you or flash with sadness, humor, shyness or anger.

During the observation period of three or four minutes, track what happened, then report it to your client. "You were here in the beginning, and then you shut down and disappeared, and seemed to recover at the end. Then you seemed more comfortable, more present. There was a shy look and sometimes a frightened look." Sometimes with direct contact we inhibit our breath. Be sure to notice your own breath and your client's, and likewise, both of your unconscious movements.

A break in contact may signal a need to withdraw. Some people need to withdraw frequently, like breathing in and out. It's a brief way of recovering ourselves as we encounter life "out there". There is nothing wrong with withdrawal unless it is chronic and inflexible. If we are to make full contact, we must be allowed to pull back, to look away momentarily, to ground, breathe easily, and feel protected and separate.

Location

If we step on a sharp stone while walking barefoot on the beach, we may cry out and hobble for a few steps. We can feel our feet under duress. Aside from moments of pain, we may have very little experience of our bodies. We may be cut off from feeling in our backs, our shoulders, and legs. Where do we locate that part of us who takes charge and claims to be us?

Where we locate ourselves somatically is a significant question. Do we think with our head or our heart? What areas of our body have we abandoned? What part of us gathers energy to itself and what somatic parts lack the consciousness to gather to itself? As a therapist you will find it valuable to assess your own predispositions in this matter. Where do you locate yourself? How do you shift your energy, or can you? Through exercises and earlier sessions with the client, where do you think the client locates herself? Where does she seem most absent? Where are the lifeless areas of her body?

EXERCISE SIX: WHERE DO YOU LOCATE YOURSELF?

Ask your client, Where do you locate yourself? After an answer repeat the question. Tell your client that you will simple repeat the question and she should say what comes to mind. When you have gathered sufficient information, ask the client "Where don't you locate yourself?" You will probably discover that your client does not like areas of his body. You need to be sensitive to issues of shame. Exploring the emotional history of the abandoned areas of our body is a valuable step toward acceptance and integration.

Chapter 10

Grounding

Our family determines how we find our ground, how we form our territory. If we do not have plenty of touching and holding, we may never be sure of ourselves emotionally, of the ground we stand on, since we cannot trust others to hold us. It's been my experience, as well as others', that people who are not held enough have a fear of falling and hold themselves stiffly away from the earth. Those who feel shame for their sexuality and dislike for their bodily responses never really hold their ground with others.

Stanley Keleman, *The Human Ground*

Being ungrounded in this world is dangerous. The invisible energy that grounds or leaves us ungrounded plays a critical role in our successful functioning. Some people appear to accompany their bodies as if riding like a parrot on their own shoulder. Other people treat their bodies like a possession, a rental horse driven over rock and hill and then abandoned to the stable. The body is attended to, exercised regularly, but the pleasure is mainly an ego experience. The rider and horse appear to be one, but there is no heart in the relationship. How can they be grounded when they are so reluctantly embodied?

To be ungrounded is to be unstable and unsupported by the very earth we walk on. We have no foundation. We are lightweights disconnected from our feeling and unrelated to others. An ungrounded person, oblivious to surroundings, trips over himself and other people's feelings. Such a person is likely to lack a sense of inner support and to suffer a loss of confidence. The ungrounded person holds too rigidly to a viewpoint or capitulates quickly to avoid conflict.

The warriors of the world, the athletes, have paid enormous attention to grounding, to establishing firm footing and balance, since it is not enough to plant oneself down like a tree. We must be able to move and stay grounded, to put down roots and pick them up again. I knew someone who found it necessary to travel frequently and made each hotel room his home. Each night he unpacked completely and placed family pictures on the bedside table. If he were a wolf, he would have declared his territory by urinating on the four corners to declare his boundaries and establish his ground. If he were a dog he would circle the place he lies down in, a magic instinctual, protective circle. To establish our territory and protective boundary is the inevitable accompaniment to grounding.

A grounded person feels she has a right to stand here, to be here, to be heard in her silence or her voice. A grounded person need not speak to be heard while an ungrounded person may talk endlessly without result. Being grounded inevitably leads to developing boundaries, allowing oneself a protective space which challenges unwanted intruders. Being grounded is the prerequisite for feeling centered and being fully in contact. And if we are loving toward others and seek peaceful relations with the life around us, the attention to boundary heightens our awareness in relationship so that we are respectful rather than intrusive. We are intrigued by the delicate interplay of closeness and distance.

How do we become so ungrounded? Growing up we may have been faced with developmental tasks that were too difficult to accomplish satisfactorily. Perhaps we learned to stand independently, for instance, but not with confidence. We came into our genital sexuality, but we were distressed. We learned to function sexually, but never with pleasure and ease, never as fully related to ourselves or our lover. Our sexual grounding is a powerful key to our being "at home" in our body. Our sexual life reflects our strengths and injuries and the functional and durable nature of our sense of self.

Grounding is quite rightly cooperating with the earth, accepting the pull of gravity and learning to do that gracefully. But we are not rooted like trees, so that I prefer to think of grounding as a function of movement, as a moving wheel that touches the earth. Grounding is about relatedness, not only the rim as it touches, but the connectedness through the spokes of the wheel. We cannot be grounded and be disconnected in our bodies. Just bringing our energy down into our feet and legs in a grounding exercise won't do. We contain polarities which must not be disowned. We reach for the sky, extending up and out, as well as root in the earth.

In so far as we refuse to relate to others, the outer world, or inner agents of our own character which remain in shadow, disowned or undeveloped, we unplug from our grounded nature. Groundedness demands that we honor the polarities in our nature. When we center ourselves in the hub of the moving wheel, we feel the edges of our being through a relaxed connectedness and enjoy for that moment a sense of wholeness which extends far beyond ourselves.

EXERCISE SEVEN: THE TREE

Gently push on your client's shoulder as he is standing to test the stability of his stance. Explaining that energy can be held captive by images, with tangible results, instruct your client to imagine himself as a tree with roots penetrating down deeply into the earth. When he says he is visualizing that, push his shoulder once more. Compare the two pushes. Usually without the tree image, the client loses balance easily. With the tree image the client becomes remarkably rooted and difficult to move.

The understanding that images bind and release energy, is a fundamental principle of a psychological body therapy. The corollary is that blocked energy locks emotionally charged images in the body. What we think matters. The images we hold consciously or lock unconsciously in our body are important. Unless we make conscious the underlying images that govern our lives, we abandon the small range of our freedom to an arbitrary unconscious mythology.

EXERCISE EIGHT: THREE STANCES

I find that some of my clients and students stand with their feet close together. They stand in a **Child's Stance,** innocent and unprotected, not taking up room and easily pushed off balance. When I point out the stance to them, they frequently take a second stance which I call the **Defensive Stance,** a wide stance which proclaims that no one can push them over without a contest. But a third stance lies somewhere in between, the **Inner Stance,** which indicates someone is lined up with himself and is allowing maximum energy to flow up from the ground into the limbs and trunk and back to earth again.

Ask the client to assume the child's stance and describe to you how the posture feels. Repeat the process with the defensive stance. Finally, ask the client, beginning with her feet closely together, to widen her stance a little at a time, until she experiences the most satisfactory alignment, an inner stance. You may want to encourage your client to write about these experiences in a therapy journal.

EXERCISE NINE: THE ALIGNED POSITION

Once the client has identified the inner stance, he is ready to try the aligned position. In this exercise I line up my client's body according to an ideal form, but my purpose is not to freeze my client into a new form. Instead I am aiming for flexibility of movement in place of rigidity. The aligned position, with toes pointing forward and feet parallel, confronts chronically held muscle and established postures and opens legs and feet energetically to greater flow. I want to establish another position kinesthetically so that the body will reorganize itself into a third position between the old and the ideal. The body can safely find its own best inner ground.

Ask your client to stand with his feet comfortably apart, and if possible, to align his knees over his feet. Then request that he bend his knees and stand like that. There is a temptation to hold the breath when trying something new. Remind him to breathe easily. After a few moments say, "Deepen your breath slightly and feel your heels against the floor."

Notice subtle shifts of your client's energy, evidenced in movements of the foot, ankle and knee. Reflect back to your client your observations. While he holds this pose for five or ten minutes, the client can tell you about experiences, images and changes he feels in his feet, ankles and legs.

EXERCISE TEN: FLEXIBLE FEET

Our feet do not move as they might were we walking barefoot on uneven surfaces of earth and rocks. Perhaps our "understanding" suffers from the loss. Certainly we have lost our surefootedness in the natural world. For this exercise you need a tennis ball, rubber ball, or a baseball. Standing, without shoes, your client rolls her foot on the ball, pressing down and feeling the bones and the tense muscles respond. These feelings can become quite pleasurable. After a few minutes, ask her to stand and feel how much more alive and in contact her feet are with the ground.

Vibration

Everything living vibrates and has a vibratory signature. A glass will vibrate at one frequency and a rock at another, so that even inanimate objects may be provoked into sound and identified and classified among the many levels constituting the "music of the spheres." Some chanted tones calm the mind and transform consciousness. For centuries many devout monks of Tibet have intoned "ohm" not only for themselves but to lift the entire energetic level of the planet. When we talk of using vibration in bodywork, we are not talking of an isolated, newly discovered phenomenon.

In our exercises, we challenge certain muscle groups in which the tissue is frozen and musculature chronically tense to increase their energetic flow. During an exercise that stresses a "frozen" area, a perceptible vibration often results, a trembling that seems to assist in energy flow.

If you stand with bent knees, for instance, soon your legs may ache. They may scream to stop. Chronically tense muscle has usually been bunched up tightly for years, a very painful experience were it not for the frozen withdrawal of energy. When such a muscle is stressed further, it awakens screaming. When you stop the exercise, the pain immediately disappears, lost once more in its death-like cloak.

A relaxed healthy muscle that tires after strenuous work does not stop aching entirely after the work ceases. A healthy muscle has no frozen retreat. The therapist must use discretion to determine whether to support the client to stay with the exercise in the face of discomfort or to rest. Vibration and full breathing leads to the free flow of energy throughout the body. We may be frightened or embarrassed at our body's trembling, but the trembling will shake us free.

EXERCISE ELEVEN: BREATHE AND BEND

Your client begins in the aligned position, with knees bent, and bends his knees further as he inhales. With each exhalation, he straightens his legs slightly. This movement confronts the chronically held muscle which deadens feeling and interrupts the energetic flow crucial to grounding. After five or ten minutes the client may feel his legs vibrate. Encourage your client to accept the vibration, as it assists in relaxing the tense muscle.

Once your client's legs vibrate, the up and down movement can be put aside. With time or good fortune, the vibration will move up the legs into the pelvis and beyond. Gradually over five sessions, as clients acclimate to the discomfort, increase the time of standing from five or ten minutes to thirty minutes. Have the client write in his journal as well as talk about the experience.

EXERCISE TWELVE: THE BEND-OVER

With the bend-over we affirm our legs and pelvis while letting go of holding in our upper body. There is a tendency to compensate for ungroundedness in the lower body by "holding on" with watchful eyes and the musculature of our arms and shoulders, as if we were grasping the outer world for safety. When our upper body relaxes, it is free to negotiate in the interactive push and pull of relationship. Assured of its support, the upper body is open to play.

In this exercise, kinesthetic awareness is developed in the spine. The exercise also opens the body to vibration and serves as a distraction from the discomfort of grounding exercises. Often in the bend-over, the therapist can observe that the client's back appears to be broken into sections. He may observe muscle bulges, flatness and irregularities. The spine may appear to dive down, disappear under flesh and emerge later. Holding in the neck is revealed in the client's inability to curl it. Instead, she holds it rigidly up and back.

Standing in the aligned position, the client begins the bend-over by curling down her head slowly, and allowing it to lead the rest of her body into a bend. If possible, she feels her back and spine, vertebra by vertebra. She notices the pull of her musculature, and finally her upper body hangs in a relaxed way. Her lower body now provides her total support. Encourage her to let go in her upper body even more with each exhale.

In addition you may observe a contraction of the neck with each inhalation and the extension with each exhalation. Ask your client to notice the movement of her head and neck with her breath. To extend the exercise, tell your client to plant her heels firmly and "walk out" on her hands to increase the stretch of the ham strings. To return to an upright position, the client uncurls slowly feeling the movement of each vertebra, the neck and head uncurling last.

EXERCISE THIRTEEN: ROCKING

Standing, the client rocks slowly forward and back, shifting his weight from the balls of his feet to his heels and back again. As he rocks back and forth slowly, instruct him to notice the shifts in balance, the muscle changes, and to test the range of his stability. Ask your client to seek a midpoint, pause there, and feel the comfort of that balanced posture. Encourage your client to feel the pulse of his breath and notice how his body can rock with each breath. The inhalation can pull the body forward slightly and the exhalation can rock the body back on its heels. This movement is subtle and needs to be initiated by the breath.

Rocking comforted us during childhood. The swaying movement can fill us with magical ease. Our muscles, paired in opposition to each other, tighten and relax like the guy ropes of a tent, and provide reflective moments of muscular integration and balance.

EXERCISE FOURTEEN: CIRCLING

Your client begins standing with her feet close together. Tell her to bring her weight forward to the balls of her feet. Then she moves the weight to the outer edge of her right foot and gradually shifts her weight back to the heel. From the right heel the weight is shifted to the left heel, the left edge of the foot and then forward to the ball of the left and then right foot. In this way, the client gradually moves her weight in a circle, feeling the outer boundaries of her feet. Circling establishes the boundaries of balance and points out breaks in our physical awareness during which we lose our balance. Usually we have a weakness in our circling perimeter where we are most likely to fall. When your client finds a place of instability, ask her to stop and hold her attention on that area, remembering to breathe easily, before she moves on. Direct the client to return to that weak spot of awareness and breathe into it. Another way to find instabilities in footing is to have the client walk extremely slowly one step at a time.

Chapter 11

Seven Stages of Grounding

The body is the best vehicle for the self caught in the particularity of time; grounding relates the self to a body moment by moment. Our grounding from birth through adulthood moves through seven stages, any of which may be flawed and unresolved.

In the first stage we are grounded on the belly of our mother and our bodies brought into conscious time by being touched by hands of love. Our bodily ego is formed horizontally first, and we make contact with our eyes and mouth as our upper body awakens. We will not contract from life if our body is welcomed and supported. If we have not been touched to the heart as children in the early stages, we will not sufficiently ground in this world. We will not feel like we have a home anywhere. We will not belong to anyone. Our egos, so presumptuous without our bodies, will not develop fluidly, nor with sufficient integration. What the mother does not touch remains undeveloped and unconceptualized, so that we grow up with impoverished images of our embodied selves.

There is a story told by Rabbi Abraham Heschel that as a youth he wondered why God had not created a temple where all the people of the world could worship. After pondering this problem for some time, he realized that God had created a temple in time, the Sabbath. In a similar way, we might wonder why Spirit remained so intangible when, for ages, people in great fervor have cried out for the manifestation of an abundant, loving God. However, even without religious belief, we may experience Spirit visible and tangible in the body. When we withdraw from the body as if it were beneath us, we lose our groundedness in Spirit. We don't believe in the body, in its beauty and its meaning down to the very edges of its form. What pleasure it is to study the body without judgement, to develop a sense of body as holy ground. If we could see the body as spiritual manifestation, we would not be at war with its aging. We would not let our vision narrow from vanity and lust. Nowhere is the manifestation of spirit as body more evident than in the devotion of a mother toward her newborn child, our first stage of grounding. Strangers are enticed to talk to young mothers, whose tender faces are lit by the fire of new life.

While the first developmental stage is horizontal, the second stage, which is as vertical, awakens the lower body. We learn to crawl, stand and walk. We develop boundaries and territory. We learn to stand up for ourselves, for a nature and identity separate from our mother. We learn as a separate being to tolerate conflict and soothe ourselves. We are curious. We learn to tumble, hop and explore. We can abandon ourselves to the adventure. We can take a stand and recover from assault.

If our separateness and healthy dependence is not supported and reflected to us in a positive light, we will struggle in relationships between merging and remaining distant, vacillating awkwardly or remaining mired in one postural polarity. The inadequacies of this grounding stage is reflected in the legs, ankles, feet, spine and how our feet plant themselves and our energy blocks. For instance, a coldness may run down our leg and weakness exist in a collapsed ankle. We might wonder "How could anyone stand for long on that leg?" For some people childhood was so unsafe that standing was painful and difficult, fraught with terror. Caught in the tissue of the adult limb is the terror of the helpless child who is trying desperately to stand prematurely and unassisted. Our awkwardness and ambivalence extends up the spine. "Why can't we stand up straight?" we ask ourselves futilely. With injuries in the second stage of grounding, it is not easy to stand up in the world as an adult.

The third grounding relates to intimate relationship and our sexuality. The second grounding had something of the centaur about it, the awakening of the powerful animal, our more primitive assertive instinctual lower half. The third grounding relates to the myth of Cupid and Psyche, the magic of divine love and the loss of love that can only be regained through terrible trial. In the third grounding the poignancy of deep love comes into greater expression as love is subjected to limitation, trial and loss. Freud understood this period in terms of the myth of Oedipus. This is a time when a child seeks the exclusive possession of one parent and fends off the other parent. The child, however, must find a way for love to survive without his exclusive ownership or control of the loved parent. When the child rejects one of his parents, he fears injury from that parent. Caught in the turmoil of ambivalent feeling, he succeeds through identification to join with his parental adversary, to become like him in some way. Without the understanding support of parents in the love triangle, a child can fail to ground his sexual identity. A child cannot lose the love of either parent without suffering psychological injury. During this stage a child often must let go of special attention from one parent to win greater independence. In our life development, each initiation to a higher level is met with a loss. We must let go of what we had before. Our third grounding was tortuous, passionate, and conflicted—a struggle protected within the family.

The fourth grounding has to do with moving from the inner family into the outer world to establish ourselves among a field of others. We enter school. In the rough and tumble of school we must survive winning and losing, intellectual and personal complexity, and retain a sense of self intact. We sit behind the wheel of an untested, powerful, strange machine, our developing body. Everything is so concrete when we are seven or eight years old. We change rules and fight over them in games. To accept mutually agreed upon rules and not revert to one's own arbitrary rule is a developmental milestone. Grounding at this stage is predominantly about what kind of losses and compromises we make to cooperate with others. This grounding of relatedness with our peers and teachers is more difficult if there was problematic grounding at the earlier stages.

71

In the fifth grounding of adolescence we move from concreteness to abstraction, from a knowable world of basic mastery to a world broken open by biological force—irrational, driven, barely contained. In the fifth grounding we move away from the family, particularly the mother, who remembers us as a child, and we join a new generation. We learn to dream great dreams. A rebellious soaring component to our nature awakens.

The story of Phaeton captures the expectation and failure of our new predicament. Phaeton in his youth was taunted occasionally by his school friends because he had no father. His mother finally told him a preposterous truth. "Your father," she said, "is the Sun." Fortunately, the Sun lived in a neighboring domain, and Phaeton, armed with his presumptuous knowledge dared to approach the fearsome blazing deity. In the face of such blinding light, Phaeton told the Sun what his mother had claimed and the god acknowledged that Phaeton was indeed his child. Like an absentee father, he immediately promised far too much. He offered to fulfill any wish his son asked, and his son, with no father to assist in developing judgement and his newly found identification with the Sun as yet unrefined, asked for more than he could handle. He wanted to drive the Sun's chariot across the sky and would not be persuaded otherwise. His dreams were inflated and unrelated to his earthbound capacities. As a result, he fatally crashed, setting the world on fire. He had had no appreciation for the consequences of his actions. It is a disturbance of this stage to be in a boundless state of imaginings, or the reverse, to be unable to dream, to act like a well-behaved little adult, to face no dangers and never risk pushing beyond our limits.

While the fifth stage of grounding is to extend, have vision, strike out for oneself, the sixth stage, young adulthood, represents limitation and restriction of reality. From identification with our godlike nature we must swing to the other polarity and deal with our earthbound fate and embodiment. Grounding can be a hard fall in the sixth stage. We must earn a living and "work for dear life." We must start small, postpone, and measure out our dreams in spoonfuls. We move into other people's jurisdictions and perhaps displace the father's authority there. The father is supposedly available to help us during adolescence, but in young adulthood we ground in a way that either cooperates with the hierarchy of the father or displaces him, rendering the older generation obsolete. We have to go past the generation we are invited into. We need acceptance and training from the older generation, and then we need to surpass them in some way. Icarus and Daedalus, his father, illustrate the failure of the sixth stage.

Daedalus the inventor, having created the maze for King Minos to contain the Minotaur, sought to escape the imprisonment of the king, who did not want to lose the irreplaceable genius of Daedalus. Daedalus constructed wings for his son and himself, using wax to attach the feathers. His son, during the escape, caught in the ecstasy of flying, failed to attend to the instructions of his father and flew too close to the sun, melted the wax, and plunged into the sea. The integration of authority, our relatedness to the past, and attention to craft are central to the grounding of the sixth stage. We must accept limitation and not sacrifice our dreams. We must accept the limitations of being single, being gay, being married with a family, and honor our commitments to others, our jobs and profession. We must allow ourselves to be ordinary and simple, trusting that what is unique in us will emerge without a struggle to be noticed.

In the seventh stage, sometimes after years of walking this planet, we let go of the earth and earthly concerns. Our love affair with the world, if we had one, no longer matters. Even the body seems an apparition because we must extend ourselves into the sky. Having firmly found our footing in the world, we legitimately seek our relatedness to a higher Nature. Of course, we are not to abandon the body for long, but rather, shift our relationship to it as we establish the priority of the inner life over the external physical world. We bring energy and rain from the blue sky down to the dusty brown earth. Because we are related to sky and earth, we live with faith. We have heart in an uncertain treacherous world. We defend an ethic of justice and love that seems to have no basis in the disillusioned view of the corrupt planet. We reach out to our full humanity and do not settle for a merely crafty, self-serving earth-bound life.

Initially in life we are sustained by a biological optimism, seemingly limitless. In our youth our bodies recover easily from each assault and inexplicably, we just feel good. But a time comes when we have no extra. Our bodies present us with all the consequences of misuse. From abundance we are thrust into limitation. It is as if we are to cross a bay in a motorboat to reach an island a distance of, say, five miles, but are only given gas for three miles. Somehow to reach that island we have to call on unexpected resources. We need faith and a courageous heart; we need to paddle with our hands, if necessary. We can no longer depend on nature to get us there. We must reach into the sky. If we can manage the inner marriage of earth and sky, people all around us will find a little haven of faith. The impossible inexplicably occurs, sometimes in contradiction to all the rules of limitation we thought as the immutable conditions of our temporal life. Finally, through the embodiment of our spiritual nature, our full groundedness is established.

Chapter 12

Boundaries

The education into the world of Self vs. Other is a process
that is completely dependent on the bodies of other people.
If it does occur in the womb, it depends on the mother, via
her "representative," the placenta. But from the time of birth,
in any case, one is envolved with the bodies of others in terms
of gesture, gaze and touch. The phenomenon of mirroring,
i.e., the growth of self-recognition through the medium of
other people.

—Morris Berman, *Coming to Our Senses*

Unless we feel grounded, it's difficult to have flexible, functioning
boundaries, and without boundaries we can count on, it's difficult
to be in contact in any consistent way. Boundaries give us protection. They also tell people where they are intruding. They give people something to bump up against, to identify who we are on a
social interactive level, and people really like to bump up against
us to find out who we are. There are some people who live in the
world as if we all drove bumper-cars. Those people who withdraw
secretly and have no external bumpers get violated quite seriously.
Children have been accused of cruelty to other kids, teasing them
relentlessly. Of course, children can be cruel, but sometimes kids
tease others to find out who they are. They push and get no response
so they push and push some more. The victimized child's healthy
retaliation may have been inhibited, and the child feels powerless.

We are all called on by others to declare who we are, what territory we command, and those of us who have abandoned our right to a certain space around ourselves find ourselves attracting more intrusive people. Perhaps only through intrusion can we establish the contact we shy away from. Some of us have been severely intruded on in childhood and have never learned appropriate boundaries. We have also developed inflexible boundaries keeping others at a distance because when we cried out in our need, our parents were not there. In our growing despair at abandonment, we grow rigid and distant, our boundaries a wall to protect us from our powerful unfulfilled hunger.

Four Circles of Space

Around each of us extends space in four successive circles: intimate, social, neutral and infinite space. Infinite space is mere background for our life encounters. The sky, mountains, and ocean are there when we lift our eyes. As infinite space approaches us, it becomes neutral space where we observe others but feel no obligation to acknowledge their presence. If I sit at an outdoor cafe watching children at play near a fountain some twenty feet away, most likely I will feel no obligation to engage them. If I don't gain their attention by staring, I am free to observe them impersonally as one might watch a movie. They are in a neutral space. Another customer at the next table is free to treat the space between us as neutral or social.

In an elevator, intended as neutral space, we can be confused by our proximity to others, because standing so close is more typical of social space where one is under pressure to nod, smile, or offer a greeting. At a closer distance we expect social engagement unless a local rule overrides the general rule, like the New Your subway rule where someone leaning against your back is still in neutral space. Usually someone physically close within the second circle of social space calls for social response. At a park, someone sits on the bench beside me. I feel restless. Is this neutral or social space? In New York and other big cities space is neutral unless you know the person. In a small town, a park bench is social space and friendly gestures are expected. Intimate, social and neutral spaces are highly variable, affected by location, culture and prior acquaintance. If someone you know is across the street, you may feel awkward not acknowledging them even if they don't see you.

Intimate space extends out usually one or two feet from our body. If people get too close to us, we may withdraw, freeze up, or attack. There are people who move from our social to our intimate space, unaware of a boundary of discomfort. They steal from us, presuming an intimacy with us by stepping through boundaries we may never have clearly established. We may be afraid to draw a line to keep some people at arm's length, at a social distance. For our purposes, the distinction between intimate and social space is crucial.

EXERCISE FIFTEEN: 360 DEGREES APPROACH

We often have radically different reactions to people as they approach us from the center, the left side, the right side and from behind. We also feel differently toward people situated below us or above us. When we feel powerless to defend our outer space from intrusion, we establish a hidden boundary within, a wall visible in the eyes.

Stand at some distance facing your client at the third circle, of neutral space, and find the boundary where social engagement begins. Your client tells you how close you can come before he feels uncomfortable. Walk slowly. Take a step and ask your client "How does this feel?" Where is the boundary that sets apart the social from the intimate space?

As therapist you must be particularly careful not to approach closer than you sense is safe for the client. The therapist is responsible to read the body language and notice the discrepancy between what the client says and the body's glance of fear, withdrawal, shallow breath, or shrug of uneasiness. In particular I study the client's eyes for evidence of the client's emotional state.

Repeat the process on the left side and the right side. The client can partially turn his head toward you but the body must be facing center. Be sure to discuss the feelings you observe with the client clarifying your observations with questions. If you notice fear in your clients eyes or body, stop and discuss what is happening. Share the observation and give the client time to reflect and to experience the feeling. Do not step closer, violating a boundary that needs to be established there.

Invariably, when I conduct this exercise in a group, no matter how sophisticated the players, people violate their own boundaries. Many people don't feel where the boundary is. They look scared. They withdraw inside themselves, but still they say "fine" instead of saying "get out of my face." Such inattention indicates how serious early violation has been by parents and others.

With children the boundaries change. We change their diapers, and then we allow them to keep the door closed when they are sitting on the toilet. At first we attend to every aspect of their being. Every decision is ours to make, but gradually we need to give over the control or we become "intrusive."

By not being sensitive to the gradations of power and space as the child grows, we fail to educate our children in a sense of personal boundary. In some families a child is not allowed to say "no" to a parent without verbal or physical abuse. A child who protests or shows anger is humiliated. How can a person believe in boundaries when their separate identity has never been respected before? The development of healthy boundaries is quite rare because it represents an education in selfhood that depends upon a special awareness by the parents.

EXERCISE SIXTEEN: NO, STAY AWAY

Stand at a distance of five or ten feet from your client, a "safe" distance. Have your client say "no." Have your client say "Stay away." Have your client say "Stay away" with his hands in front of him as if to push you away. Explore the distance between you. Study your client's body and face for evidence of fear, anger or playful confidence. Reflect back your observations after you have asked your client about his emotional response to the exercises. Gradually move closer repeating the exercise, noting the differences. You can with some client's have them push against you using a pillow as a buffer. Without a clear no, we cannot have a clear yes.

On a body level, at the very least, we should be able to keep the world at arm's length, but I often find people unwilling to command the space between their own chest and their arm's extension. Here, at the very least, the boundary should be set. To keep the world at arm's length, to push people away with our arms, is a critical aspect of our healthy development. We need to believe in the power of our arms to protect us. By learning our boundaries, we can then truly welcome others in.

Chapter 13

Breathing

Breathing is the self; without it life does not exist. Yet, para-
doxically, life resides in the silence, the brief pause between
inspiration and expiration. With this pause the healthy person returns over and over to his original being and rests anew
in his self. This pause is a core, a center of power, a source
that nourishes and sustains. I shall call it the unconscious,
spiritual self. To find one's true "self" is to be able to return
to this original state, to return to the promising silence.

Lillemor Johnsen, *Integrated Respiration Theory/Therapy*

Everything alive pulsates and vibrates. The pulse may be too slow
for us to notice in a tree and the vibration too fast in a leaf. Unaware
of the pulse and vibration of nature, we are unlikely to notice pulse
and vibration in ourselves. Even without a stethoscope we can feel
the indefatigable pulse of our hearts and marvel at how they slow
and seemingly falter or speed up, so relentless and so variable. Like
a bird in a cage, the heart speaks of life beyond its confines. A second pulse pumps cerebral spinal fluids, a deep, secret stream of life,
through the spine and brain. And more fully expressive as a rhythm
is breathing, which feeds the cells with new life.

Like the beating of our heart and the contractions of our intestines, our breath functions independently of our consciousness:
an unconscious function which establishes a basic body rhythm,
a pulse of energy like a wave that peaks and recedes across our body
ocean. When we were young our rib cage was vibrant and flexible,

and our ribs as they joined our spine at our back moved easily and quite visibly with each breath, mimicking an accordion expanding and contracting. With such full and natural breathing our bodies maintained a high energy level, easily flushed from head to toe with anger or excitement, were open to love and pain alike. And with each breath our pelvis tilted forward and swung back, and our neck and head moved. Our shoulders shifted with each breath and our nose and mouth mysteriously varied its shape and trembled slightly. Breath symbolizes the raw force and vitality of life energy, like ocean breakers manifesting the power of the sea.

Over time, our full breath has been reduced, our ribs grown inflexible, the pulse dimmed, our sea of energy thrown into an enforced and chilling calm. With diaphragm tightened, our breath does no longer reaches down to our genitals, no longer connects the upper and lower body. How have we suppressed our life energy?

Reich informs us that holding our breath and contracting our diaphragm are early mechanisms we use to suppress sensations of anxiety and pleasure. Reich came to the conclusion that anxiety had its seat in the respiratory and cardiac system. When we experience anxiety, frequently we feel it in our chest and diaphragm. Anxiety can be experienced in other body areas, such as the abdomen, as well.

For many years Freud had described anxiety as transformed libido, as wine turns to vinegar, but in 1926, Freud redefined anxiety as an ego function, as a signal of danger, as a response to the feared loss of the object (originally, the mother), as fear of castration turned to moral and social anxiety in the shadow of the superego's presence. Reich believed that Freud's earlier ideas about anxiety were correct, that dammed up libidinal energy was experienced as anxiety. Libidinal energy is experienced as pleasure when it moves from the core of the body to the periphery; during contraction, energy moves from the periphery into the body's core and is experienced as anxiety.

Reich paid particular attention to breathing while working with clients. Since respiration was a measure of neurotic holding, patients were not to force breathing, but were to breath naturally and deeply.

Particularly in the exhalation, he found clients holding back. During the exhalation Reich applied gentle pressure with his fingers between the sternum and umbilicus. His contact coupled with deep breathing resulted in the relaxation of the abdominal wall. Reich would ask his clients to "give in" completely. With deep expiration Reich found the patient in an attitude of surrender. The head moves back, the shoulders gently forward, the abdomen gathers in, the pelvis pushes forward and the legs open.

Breathing is an energetic pulsation that transforms the whole body. Reich's deep uninhibited breathing of surrender leads to the orgasm reflex, the involuntary energetic release of the entire organism. Without full respiratory release, the upper body, the seat of anxiety and the center for three powerful pulses (heart, breath, and cerebral spinal pulse), stands against the lower body, the pelvis, the seat of instinctual energies. Reich in 1935, working with a patient to release dammed up libidinal energies to bring about a full orgastic release, triggered the orgasm reflex, the instinctual pulse of the lower body. The reflex was evidence of energetic streaming and bodily surrender in Reich's "character-analytic vegetotherapy," later to be called "orgone therapy."

Reich's technical plan was to find where the inhibition to the orgasm reflex located itself and to intensify that inhibition. Contracting a muscle, "breathing into it" or massaging the area were methods that increased the experience of the inhibition prior to its release. In response the body seeks out the natural path for the excitation. Reich noted that when holding dissolved in the neck, the throat, and chin, his client felt the impulse in the chest and shoulders only to then shut it down by an inhibiting response. After the inhibition in the client's chest was interrupted, the impulse and his contraction against it located themselves in the abdomen. This process naturally led Reich to work with the upper body before working to release energy in the pelvis.

Influenced by Reich's work, Lillemor Johnsen grew interested in the undeveloped muscle, the areas seemingly ignored in a system studying the release of contracted muscle. The hypotonic muscle, Johnsen feels, holds resources and repressed material which

83

can be awakened through attention to "the breathing wave," a pulsation travelling through the entire body. Lightly touching areas of the body, the therapist can feel the tonus of the muscle and also feel the energetic movement responsive to the breath.

EXERCISE SEVENTEEN: STAND AND BREATHE

Ask the client to stand, close her eyes, deepen her breath slightly. Attend to the rhythm of her breathing. Notice how her body begins to shift with each inhalation and exhalation. Notice movement in the pelvis and any other part of the body and ask your client to exaggerate the movements slightly. The client allows her body to shift to establish a rhythmic movement responsive to her breath.

EXERCISE EIGHTEEN: BREATHING LYING DOWN

Your client lies down on a bed or comfortable rug with knees up and feet flat on the floor. Direct him to breathe naturally and notice in a five minute period all the sensations and feelings that emerge. Write down what you notice about his breath and body response. Do not intrude on the client by touching or demanding a response. The client needs time to sink into his body's rhythms and let go of the demands of the outer world. Watch to see if your client is able to relax. How does he hold back from the surrendering to his internal rhythms?

Does the client labor through the inhalation or restrict the exhalation? Is there a restful pause between inhaling and exhaling? If the client forces the inhalation and is confused by your suggestion to breathe naturally, suggest to him that he not take the next breath. Let his body breathe him. The client is to wait for his body to grab the next breath out of the stillness of his being there.

You may suggest that your client deepen his breath if it seems extremely shallow. There may be areas of his upper body that appear grey and lifeless, without much energy compared to other areas. You may find it useful to hold your hand a few inches above the deadened area or even to touch the area. Obviously, such choices depend on the client's development, your training, and the transference and countertransference considerations.

EXERCISE NINETEEN: LOOSENING THE DIAPHRAGM

You are to explore with your client a more artificial breath process which divides the inhalation into two actions. Your client starts to inhale filling up her chest. Midway through the inhalation, direct your client to "kick" the breath down into her belly as she completes the in breath. This loosens the diaphragm. The client exhales in one gesture.

Most of us tend to be either chest breathers or belly breathers; one form comes more easily than the other. With this exercise, we switch from a chest to belly breath and this shift facilitates the energetic connection between chest and belly.

Section Three

Character and Restructuring

Chapter 14

Character and Character Armor

I wander thro' each chartered street,
Near where the chartered Thames does flow,
And mark in every face I meet
Marks of weakness, marks of woe.

William Blake, "London"

Having explored the foundations for contact in the second section, stressing in particular the development of kinesthetic awareness, we are prepared in Section Three to address the issues of character and character armor. We discuss the five character types established by Alexander Lowen to evaluate character as emotional attitude and body armoring. The character types also give us a way to direct our realignment. As a further aid to restructuring, I have provided eight stations of the body-standing-up.

The first tasks of an analytic psychotherapy are to identify the client's false self (character) that developed in childhood to adapt to the world and to help the client differentiate him or herself from the principal caretakers. The second task is to meet the unconscious. In a somatic analysis we study the postural set of the body, the gestures, unconscious movement and the underlying images that bind and release energy. We help the client differentiate his or her core body nature from rigid defenses and incorporated body images. We also meet the unconscious body with gentle attention, attuning to and evoking its pulse.

The Unrecovered Body

In shadow our bodies are a mystery, an uncultivated, largely unexplored wilderness, with plains and mountain ranges, deserts, uncharted rivers, and brilliant night skies. In shadow our unrecovered bodies hold the marks of earlier misfortunes. When we can read the body's story, a history consciously unfolds which would not be available to us otherwise. The body as shadow includes the character we developed, the body manifestations of our inner yearnings, and the repressed and the unexplored unconscious. While recognizing the breadth and mystery present in the body as shadow, we will focus here on character in order to differentiate the false self from our core nature.

It is far easier to identify character than to identify our core nature. What is true about us is most illusive, most unique, and, in a fortunate therapy, is sensed and known in the intimacy between therapist and client.

Certainly the therapeutic persona does not contact the deep nature of our clients. The therapeutic persona sets the rules and knows the game of therapy, but the therapist's professional disguise can also be a false self, diffusing genuine response with imitations of concern, a paint by numbers approach to therapy.

Our task is interpersonal as well as intrapsychic. In short term work, we can resolve crisis as "the therapist." But in long term therapy, only genuine presence and true contact brings forth the deep healing of our injured humanity. We are moved by our client's being. We are drawn forth into our vulnerability and we speak from our heart. There is no technique, no clever use of words, and no substitute for the intuitive nature stepping forth as human soul. The competent professional identifies character, but only the person of the therapist meets the client's core nature.

Posture as Character

The posture we develop from childhood may be belligerent, indifferent, passive, attentive, ingratiating, aloof, shy. In some way a chilling reduction of life to something repetitive and familiar, our posture represents a severe cramping of our early life force by which we block the flow of energy in our body and deaden feeling. Prolonged contraction of muscle and other tissue is so painful that we find a way selectively to "freeze" body sensation. Character, no matter how aggressive in style, is passive, an artful, lifeless withdrawal. Our numbing passivity, a response to trauma, reduces both the frightening and the miraculous to the mundane and trivial. As a posture, character discounts the present moment through a repetitive, egocentric indifference to life.

In the Bible, when Jesus was fatigued by the demands of others, he sought refuge in the wilderness to pray. His active distancing was not the passive withdrawal of character. He entered the inner wilderness, to drink undisturbed from the well of Spirit that penetrates to the foundations of life. Stepping back to renew our energy is not the frozen mechanical withdrawal of character built on unrelatedness.

Analytic psychology argues that early relationships condition our later responses. We establish our identity by being acknowledged and emotionally supported as children. If unloved and unseen, we may cling to our mother or father, depending on the parent, rather than trusting to stand on our own legs. Identifying with the good and ill in our parents, we carry their burdens, fears, hates, and unfulfilled lives as our own. We are sponges indiscriminately soaking up the life around us. We smoke their cigarettes and sip from their drinks left over from the night before. We posture to please and assure our survival but our mask leaves our vital nature unaddressed.

Our posture holds all the elements of our compromise hidden within us. Our posture expresses our attitude which may be the underlying, organizing image of our functional life. We may have a "bad attitude" that, in fact, has sustained and protected us through hard times. The analytic task is to identify the attitude, the underlying images, the posture and its represented compromises, and help the client differentiate herself from early identifications. In the body's recovery we free up vital energies and awaken new attitudes. Our illnesses and injuries inform us. We study the shadow in its range and depth, not to make us wrong but to make us whole.

Character Armor, the Embodied Lie

When I grew up, character was considered a good thing. If someone had character, it meant he had been through a few tussles in the world. He'd not won them all, only a fair share, and he survived with some quality of inner strength, some ethical, inner victory in defeat. Character stood for the gains of age, the wisdom of one who has journeyed through time for a spell without selling out friends and family.

The purely negative meaning of the Reichian "character" robs us of these precious connotations which most of us in the trade relinquish too quickly. Character to the Reichian means a rigid, maladaptive, repetitious response to the world developed as a defensive action during an earlier life trauma, a response which inhibits our somatic and psychic repertoire, collecting debris on the psyche-soma levels like a log jam in a stream. The study of character is not then the study of the nobleness of great men and women, but the study of defensive behaviors so unindividual as to be duplicated in great numbers of people. Whereas one might imagine a person of character to be unique, the Reichian character speaks of the most boring, unrewarding aspect of our nature, and its body analog, character armor.

Often in response to stress and trauma, our body tenses and muscles contract. We hold our breath in momentary fright, but afterward we do not always relax completely. Our shoulders tighten with rage, but we dare not strike our parents. Our shoulders continue to hold the rage through the years as our muscles, once contracted, refuse to extend. The tight muscle aches initially until we replace the pain with numbness. With the loss of feeling, we lose critical somatic feedback, so that years later we may dangerously stress our back, for instance, because we cannot feel the warning signs of pain. As a result, our body becomes less tolerant of high energy which would disturb contracted areas. A frozen area develops a "thermostat," maintaining energy at unthreatening levels. A diffuse anxiety persuades us to stay within energy parameters, to maintain frightened, upraised shoulders and a compliant smile.

Character armor is the way the body tolerates a contradiction in tissue, a lie in structure. Those of us who have suffered early trauma employ the most primitive defenses of denial, projection, introjection and splitting. Our desperate rejection of feeling and our inability to integrate the shadow, our split away from dark rages and incestuous desires are facilitated by body numbness and our splitting off from bodily awareness. Our bodies reflect the violence of these early childhood injuries.

Identity and Individuation

The accommodation we make in childhood is often under duress. I think of the character we adopt as similar to awakening to a fire in the middle of the night and grabbing what is near at hand to cover ourselves outside. One person wears only a blanket hastily bunched over the shoulders and another wears a tee shirt and underwear. Whatever we have taken in haste becomes enshrined as our "nature." We have no way of "knowing" that our immobilized thick shoulders have warded off psychic blows and held back rage. We do not know that we have adopted our mother's slouch, her despair, and our father's stride with the weight riding back on the heels. And we will never know unless we pursue a somatic analysis in which our body structure is observed and challenged. It is character, of course, that has compromised the foundations of contact. Character has weakened our boundaries, ungrounded us, constricted our breathing, and swallowed our feeling. As we build flexible boundaries and relatedness, we feel the pulse of our core nature and move with grace.

Jung believed that as human beings we innately sought our own growth which he called individuation. Jung saw our society as sick, and therefore being well adapted was not advantageous. When people developed symptoms of emotional disorder, he felt that the symptoms represented a healthy outcry, a movement toward health.

We have through character reduced the world to bite size. Through egocentricity we have excluded key aspects of life, and sometimes with our over simplified model, survived quite successfully for a while, until we developed "symptoms."

Whatever our fantasies have been concerning who we are, our identity has left footprints in the past. Perhaps we catch a glimpse of our true nature in a vision of our future. As we work to clear ourselves of false identities, we find ourselves more vulnerable and alive, no longer protected by fictions whose sole purpose was to comfort at the price of blindness. We live more on the cutting edge of our life with no time to rehearse, a life without the deadened predictability of the past. We are, through the body-psyche's individuation, in a world more trustworthy and spontaneous where reality is more clearly distinguished from fantasy.

The blurring of fantasy and reality is essential to the embodied lie of character. To liberate our imagination from misuse relieves the body of a terrible burden. The body cannot distinguish the truth from the lies we tell it. If we imagine a terrible threat to us, even though we are walking down a safe street, our body cowers and sweat drips suddenly from our armpits. A pretended life creates stress and ill health. If we are to be ill, then let the illness serve the purposes of our self development. Pain, like death, is a great teacher. And as we individuate, the great teachers come to us, and we clear the body self of fabrication.

Chapter 15

Character as Archetype

> What one has to negotiate some sort of alliance with is the patient's *practice of self-cure,* which is rigidly established by the time he reaches us. To treat this *practice of self-cure* merely as resistance is to fail to acknowledge its true value for the person of the patient. It is my belief from my clinical practice that very few illnesses in a person are difficult to handle and cure. What, however, is most difficult to resolve and cure is the patient's practice of self-cure.
>
> M. Masud R. Khan, "Towards an Epistemology of Cure"

Character provides a meeting place for psyche and soma. Character as a defense structure gathers us when we are scattered and organizes us into an identifiable pattern of rigidity and energetic withdrawal, binding our anxiety, rage, sadness and longing. Character is what keeps us separate, exempt and special, and what holds us back from the surrender to our energetic nature. Character represents a practice of self-cure, an ongoing, hasty, rigid solution imposed over our instability to maintain an intact sense of self. Daily our anxiety persuades us not to relinquish our protections.

Typically, when character establishes itself in a growing organism, it disrupts and inhibits the scheduled somatic function, so that muscle remains flaccid and unresponsive. With our diaphragm contracted and the ribs gripped with fear, we may never establish a pattern of full breathing. We may never develop coordinated movement between the left and right side. We may never stand up and walk in a natural easy way. Character is the shell that energy leaves behind, and as such it provides a house; but the shell, as we grow, becomes too small.

I have come to value Lowen's five characters, as distinct from those in the Diagnostic and Statistical Manual, as representing basic ego adaptations of early childhood, each with its corresponding physical characteristics. As archetypes, they are patterns of behavior that are discovered rather than invented. The spiralling structure formed as a crystal on a string suspended in water is such an example. The crystal is merely a representative of the spiralling archetype that takes other forms in nature.

Archetypes are the underlying symbolic language that different cultures adapt but do not substantially change. Arising spontaneously throughout the world, mythological motifs are common to all human nature, and represent typical and instinctive modes of impulse, thought and action. Archetypes have about them a provocative potentiality that draws us into a drama, a reenactment of inevitable patterns of response. There is never just a tree, but earth and roots and birds, as a particular story unfolds. And so with character, the form is never in isolation but creates a world within and around itself.

Character is a brief drama of adaptation with projected villains and heroes. Under pressure the child has only a few possible ways to jump. To avoid full contact the schizoid character withdraws, the oral collapses, the psychopath pretends, the masochist endures and the rigid competes. Frequently on the developmental journey, people take on more than one character. Reich had hoped that character defense could be entirely dissolved, replaced by genital character, but our early character layers, even when "worked through," remain to some degree, indelibly printed on our nature.

Reich understood character as biology. For years Reich studied contraction, expansion, tension and release in single celled organisms. He imagined how a cell might "feel" under tension. Our sexual arousal and release was functionally identical to the expansion and division in cells. The Orgasm Formula became the Life Formula. In the complex structure of man, Reich viewed the primitive tube from mouth to anus as the link to simple natural forms. We experience pleasure in expansion and anxiety in contraction. If we cannot release because of masochistic character, we are held at that perilous point, analogous to a time in a cell's life when the internal pressure of increasing fluids threatens to burst the contracting cell wall.

Character as frozen movement imposes a protective limitation, which is not necessarily bad. Limitation is the foundation of embodiment. It gives us focus and direction. Character as limiting and therefore, directing, can be seen as positive. The schizoid character who holds back from the bond of relationship may pour heart and soul into music, art, literature or science. Limitlessness, an attribute of God, must be overcome in order to function in an amazing, otherwise overwhelming, universe.

We need not conclude that the absence of character condemns us to a limitless world. Character is what keeps us from full contact with life and from energetic release. We have a core being that makes choices, a genital nature that Reich considered "good." Because character imposes an arbitrary direction, often in contradiction to our core nature, it can destroy us unless we break through the rigidity. The ungrounded psychopath cannot sustain what he or she creates. The schizoid artist may die young, be incapable of forming relationships, feel unappreciated, or find oblivion in addiction.

In an analytic bodywork that respects developmental theory, it is often useful to work from the later injuries to the earlier ones, addressing our rigid and masochistic features before our oral and schizoid qualities. Reich, in his insistence on working from the ocular segment toward the pelvis, followed a similar process by which the deep feeling of the pelvis was not tampered with until a path was cleared for the energy radiating from the vegetative center to stream through.

Before entering into an historical and theoretical discussion of character structure, I must speak of how my own character structure revealed itself to me in and out of therapy. We must value the tools we have, without presuming to think that we control the therapy. Every theoretical system hawks its wares swearing to its unique efficacy, but truly it is the insistence of our core nature that leads us through darkness to light. Gradually our inner director conducting the therapy reveals the levels and brings our focus to a potential feeling point of change.

In my own body therapy, after an initial anxious, paranoid attention toward my therapist, I worked on my predisposition to endure, the build-up in my upper back, the masochistic layer. The masochism was an overlay on a psychopathic structure in which I held on to a hard won autonomy and denied my dependency needs. Through grounding exercises and efforts to break down the defensive structure in my chest and open up my breathing, I was able to feel and express my needs, my orality. After I found my footing and could feel my legs with their strength, weakness and pain, I was able to move to the later oedipal issues and integrate feeling in my pelvis.

I was fortunate in working with a kind and gifted therapist who tracked energy, insisted on structural change and understood character structure. And yet, the year after I finished therapy I came into my schizoid nature, that part of me that withdrew from relationship, a character in direct contradiction to my oral idealism about love and loyalty to friends. That schizoid character was in collusion with my energized psychopathic manner of gathering acquaintances, and was at odds with my genital longing. I had no deep feeling access to the schizoid level until the other character structures had been addressed. In therapy we can observe our process. We can provoke or cooperate with it. We can do little more. The intellectual ego may toy with an issue but only the self discloses in its own good time.

I was in France on vacation with my wife and two year old son when I suddenly remembered a friend of my family sexually molesting me. He was gently eager for me to suck his penis. Out of the darkness of being ignored by my parents, I was delighted and quite chatty over this coveted attention. The molester heard someone coming. "Shut up or I'll kill you," he said placing his hand over my mouth. With no further explanation, he never touched me again and I mourned the loss of him. I suspect that I had been around two years old, and so my own son triggered the memory. The memory unlocked a dark key to my family, a key I had felt perfectly able to deal with years earlier. Yet, the memory had not come to me then.

The experience taught me how little control we have over the progress of therapy. It was only years later through character work related to addiction that I was able to heal early splits that had carried and caused so much pain. It seemed that only through the grace of God and the tenacity of the few people who truly loved me that I was to reach to the depth of my early injury. As therapists we are not dealing with mechanical toys accessible with a screwdriver of therapy. We may often find ourselves as no more than witnesses to a drama whose direction as a force of nature falls upon us like a birth outside our control and understanding.

Reich was able to describe character as a defense structure. He was able to identify the borderline structure in his first book, *The Impulsive Character* in 1925. In *Character Analysis* (1933) he identified the phallic narcissist, the passive feminine, the hysteric, the compulsive, the aristocratic, the masochistic, the mass, neurotic and genital characters. Freud's failure to cure masochism seemed to Reich to be one reason Freud adopted the death instinct and warned against excessive therapeutic ambition. Reich felt that he had cracked the masochistic code. He felt the death instinct was an unfortunate fabrication, a theory justifying a failure.

Reich adopted Freud's libidinal ladder with its emphasis on genital function. Behaviors traceable to pregenital organization were considered inferior adaptations, damming up libidinal energy needed for full genital functioning. Reich's theory that all neurosis is caused through damned up libido was a more inclusive statement than Freud's which held to the toxicological theory applicable to actual neurosis alone.

In step with the libidinal ladder model, Lowen's five characters progress toward the highest development of the rigid character, a nearly genital organization. The "drive model" (the repression of instinctual drives) anchored in biological development provides the natural ground for psyche and soma to meet. On the level of psyche, if we choose, we can fold in Object Relations theory, Self Psychology and Analytic Psychology, without detracting from the clarity and functional nature of the five characters.

Lowen felt that the character that formed around developmental arrests could be identified and read for its psychological and somatic content. The characters we discuss here are: the schizoid, the oral, the psychopathic, the masochistic and the rigid. Lowen amended the psychopathic character in his book *Narcissism: Denial of the True Self,* (1983) to include the range of narcissistic expression. Lowen describes five types in an order of increasing narcissism: phallic-narcissistic character, narcissistic character, borderline personality, psychopathic personality, and paranoid personality.

The schizoid, the oral and the psychopathic form a group representing early childhood damage. Between early and later damage I like to imagine a bridge (named in honor of Margaret Mahler of course) that leads us on one side from our oneness with the mother to the other side, our separateness, and that the illusion of omnipotence sustained in the merged psychopathic structure crosses over the bridge to the crushed protest and brokenness of the masochistic child on the other side. How difficult to step down as a young god joined to the power of the mother to find oneself small and powerless, shamefully driven to endure the domination of adults. The rigid character follows then as a negative adaptation to the Oedipal conflict. Failure to master genitality throws us back into an anal, masochistic mode.

The Schizoid Character

Since schizoid conditions constitute the most deep-seated of all psychopathological states, they provide an unrivaled opportunity for the study not only of the foundations of the personality, but also of the most basic mental processes.... Contrary to common belief, schizoid individuals who have not regressed too far are capable of greater psychological insight than any other class of person, normal or abnormal—

a fact due, in part at least, to their being so introverted (i.e., preoccupied with inner reality) and so familiar with their own deeper psychological processes....

W. Ronald D. Fairbairn, *Psychoanalytic Studies of the Personality*

It should come as no surprise that injury begins in the uterus, and that the attitudes toward mothering, the traumas endured by the mother, her diet and life conditions all have bearing on the baby's vitality and sense of being wanted. In many places in the United States today, the mother finds little support for what is, in fact, a life and death experience. In a culture where most young adults move and leave their childhood families, where families themselves are strained to breaking, there is little support for the mother, or the primary caregiver, and baby. Small wonder then that a baby's very existence may be threatened, not by a vicious, uncaring woman but by an exhausted, depleted woman with no place to turn. Infants, even those with a good temperamental match with the caregiver, can be difficult to provide for. After all, hospitals have three shifts of workers daily, to care for babies. The complexity of a full motherhood might once have been passed on gracefully from one generation to another, but who educates the lonely young woman in her apartment in the city? How can the tender bond be supported in a culture that is so cold-hearted to the most vulnerable of us?

The young mother who is fully present with her child does not function from instinct alone. Nature does not guarantee an intact sense of self. Good mothering is learned. Winnicott's concept of good-enough mothering frames in the minimal demand of the mother-infant relationship, but the full demand of motherhood is often exhausting. When the bottom drops out of a mother who has nothing more to give, who was inadequately mothered herself, or if the infant is difficult, ill, or hard to nurture, then frightening results can happen. The child grieves, the child rages, the child despairs, sometimes the child dies. The child's very existence is at stake. The child is not held in the loving heart of the mother. Perhaps the child is feared, misunderstood, resented or hated as an unwanted burden. Perhaps the child's helpless dependence terrifies the mother with bitter feelings of her own thwarted dependence.

A baby in the first few months lying on its back or stomach, unable to turn over by itself, has no life apart from the mother. How can such a baby grow up to form relationships if the baby experiences a desolate aloneness, and bonding means to feel the pain and rage associated with the mother? The good and bad object never come together. The child retreats away from the outer world and away from forming relationship. On the dark end of this spectrum lives a psychotic core, a pre-object state where relief comes from fragmentation and withdrawal. Life is survived, not enjoyed. Action is willed rather than felt.

Somewhere in the vast spectrum of inadequate care, the bad-enough parent tortuously maintains the child in a desolate anxiety for a long time. This is the theorized beginning for the schizoid character; however, it is unlikely that environment is always to blame. There are genetic factors that may render an infant anxious, deserted and distraught, leaving decent parents powerless to intervene. The schizoid character experiences an inward withdrawal, and a sense of a cohesive self never forms. The ego has vast functional gaps, body contact is severely reduced and thinking dissociates from feeling. Energetically bodily life withdraws to the core. The body does not connect to itself as a whole: the head, arms and legs do not extend from the trunk, nor the upper to the lower body , or the left to the right side. The hands, face, genitals and feet tend to be cold.

If you look at a person with schizoid character, you are likely to see a narrow contracted body and a mask-like face. The eyes do not make contact. There is severe holding around the eyes, through the diaphragm and all the joints. I have known people with this structure who were quite athletic. Perhaps genetically they were able to connect and coordinate adequately in spite of early trauma. Perhaps they sought out exercise as a route to feeling in spite of their numbness. I have known highly intelligent and perceptive people with schizoid character; despite their gifts life tends to be hard for them because at rest, they are not content within themselves. No one said to them "what a cute little baby" spontaneously one billion times full of love and feeling, or, if it had been said, for some reason it was not received. Nothing really makes up that difference. One must settle for the gradual development of supportive rituals to stand against the childhood memories of terror and loss. Sometimes the schizoid character underlies later developmental arrests, which resolve to reveal the earlier character.

Schizoid characters do not bond. They withdraw rather than attach. In marriage they are passive, allowing themselves to be coerced into shared activity while remaining partially aloof. In every situation they find an escape route. They will not be accountable. They will not commit. Yet, they cannot tolerate rejection and loss. The schizoid person feels essentially unlovable. They have no right to take up space on the planet. An irrational inner critic, perhaps a vicious internalized voice of mother or father, tells them they are hopelessly at fault in some way, clumsy, ugly, awkward or stupid, nothing but trouble. These negative conclusions are unshakeable. You can pour love in with a bucket and the effect, if any, lasts for an hour. They don't feel safe entertaining a positive feeling about themselves. In compensation for feelings of inferiority, they will often harbor a secret superiority. They will not be manipulated by praise into personal exposure; they turn gold into shit. If they feel envy about the therapist's office, the therapist's life real or imagined, or even the therapist's air of contentment, they may not volunteer this information. As a therapist we do not feel cared for by schizoid personalities, although some of these clients are unfailingly polite.

Some schizoid clients may instill a sense of anger and hopelessness in the therapist. The therapist will be criticized for any enthusiasms or optimistic expressions. When the client does not feel numb, he will seem fragile because any of the therapist's insights may insult him, demean him, and provide him more evidence, spoken or unspoken, of how insensitive the therapist is. These clients have no skin. Every nerve is raw. Some clients, with so little internal glue and protection, are dominated by fears of disintegration and prohibit any intervention. With some clients, the therapist will be in a bind. The therapist may be afraid to do nurturing, supportive work because any regression leads to severe anxiety, while trying to strengthen ego functioning is met with resentment as an unsympathetic demand to "get it together." The therapist may be in for months of negative transference.

Some people with the schizoid character are visionary. Their freedom from being bound by the ties of the world opens their eyes and hearts to intellect, imagination, creativity, God. Their personal needs are transmuted. They work brilliantly and passionately. And in others the schizoid structure may underlie more prominent character. They make friends and express caring but another, deeper aspect withdraws. The person may appear more convincingly as an oral, psychopath, masochist or a rigid, but underneath layers of defense lies the earliest injury.

My own tendency with schizoid issues is to proceed carefully, supporting work that develops kinesthetic awareness and integrates splits. Initially I work with the body-standing-up, employing the fundamentals of contact, to build grounding, sensing boundaries, to open up breathing and access to feeling. The schizoid does not trust outer boundaries and has withdrawn within walled fortresses behind the eyes. The therapist must work with the ocular segment to achieve a genuine visual contact. The energetic level must not be pumped up with deep breathing, because no good is achieved when a client is overwhelmed, a state which breaks the conscious awareness of self and other. Instead, the therapist constantly checks to see if the client is present and can express feeling. Very gradually the energetic level is raised by staying on the threshold of sustainable contact with the client. With opening and gathering strength, the client may stumble upon early body memories of physical, sexual and verbal abuse that traumatized him as a young child. These incidents need time to be integrated. Countertransference and transference issues must be addressed with meticulous attention throughout, or the therapist will be swept into the inner world of the client without much external reference.

The Oral Character

> ... it becomes evident that the emotional conflict which
> arises in relation to object-relationships during the early oral
> phase takes the form of the alternative, 'to suck or not to
> suck,' i.e. 'to love or not to love.' This is the conflict under-
> lying the schizoid state. On the other hand, the conflict which
> characterizes the late oral phase resolves itself into the alter-
> native, 'to suck or to bite,' i.e. 'to love or to hate.' This is the
> conflict underlying the depressive state. It will be seen, accord-
> ingly, that the great problem of the schizoid individual is how
> to love without destroying by love, whereas the great prob-
> lem of the depressive individual is how to love without de-
> stroying by hate. These are two very different problems.
>
> W. Ronald D. Fairbairn, *Psychoanalytic Studies of the Personality*

There are many good reasons why a mother is unable to be present for her child in the first year of life. She may have to go back
to work and place the child with someone else. She may have other
young children that divide her attention. The age of mother bash-
ing is over. Motherhood is extremely difficult, as difficult as creating a successful, long-term marriage. And what may seem like a
reasonable amount of attention for one child may simply be insufficient for another. Sometimes, it is true, the father and mother are
selfish, shallow people with nothing to give insisting on distance
from everyone and breaking the child's heart. Whatever the reason, with the oral character the child prematurely loses the mother
and painfully grieves and longs for her return. She is never home.
She does not hold the child for long periods. The baby-sitter reli-
giously watches TV.

Abandonment and loss that remains unresolved characterizes
this structure. The oral person loves and wants to be loved. Such
a person grows up needy, clinging, and wanting to be held and
supported, desires often thinly disguised with a veneer of independence. Underneath a warm engaging smile may be an angry
demand, a sense of entitlement. Energetically, oral types have trou-

ble sustaining tasks. They give up easily and need encouragement. They want the therapist to stand up for them. With a lower body that tends to be weak, grounding exercises are painful. They actually avoid autonomy by being ungrounded. An oral type's eyes may be weak, their feet thin, their knees locked and their upper body collapsed at the diaphragm,(station five). Their energy is kept low through shallow breathing.

The oral type often swings between elation to depression. What they look for in therapy is someone to save them, to be the mother they never had, and when the therapist fails, they are angry and biting. It is easy as a therapist to take the bait of praise and excitement as the oral character sets the hook in the narcissistic structure of the therapist. If the client is empty, the therapist surely thinks she can fill this poor client up. Marriages can happen this way: the illusion of love and of an independent free thinking mate by our side. But we find only an angry, demanding child. "Where's my dinner?" "I thought you were going to get a better job." In bed, the oral character wants comfort more than sex. They live life as though the miracle solution is always around the corner.

As a therapist we need to point out the oral pattern as it occurs. For instance, the false hopes that sets up the therapist rather than the client to perform. We need to encourage the client to ground, to endure the pain in the legs and not quit too soon. We build autonomy gently. We question entitlement. We direct the client to the unresolved feelings of loss of the mother that causes him or her to recreate childhood in all relationships and make demands that are not willingly met by healthy adults. Oral types must let go of childhood and accept limitation. They must plow and plant their own field rather than someone else's. They become co-dependents easily. The oral person may exercise the tyranny of weakness. They may express anger and disappointment at the failure of the world to hold them as special. What events in childhood taught them to collapse rather than fight? The kindness and firmness of the therapist provides a safe container for building independence and strength.

Because the oral structure suffers injury in the area of love, these types can rise to great heights in their commitment to unconditional love as an ideal, loving others while feeling unnourished themselves. Beneath the mask of weakness and need, they may have powerful reserves. A woman client, severely disappointed in a love interest, was plunged into a depression that fully reflected her childhood pain of emotional neglect. She felt the futility of all her efforts to be in satisfying relationship with a man. A few nights later, while getting out of her car, she was mugged. She felt a man push her into the car and grab her purse. She held on and struggled. Finally the man hurt her sufficiently so that she let go of the strap, but as soon as he ran, she screamed, "Stop him. He stole my purse!" Others chased him, but he managed to escape. For the two weeks following, she was showered with love and attention. All the people who knew her rallied around and she felt as if for the first time in her daily life she was profoundly loved. More importantly, she could not overlook the courage and power that erupted spontaneously within her when she was attacked. The mugging and its aftermath proved a turning point in this woman's work regarding her oral structure.

The Psychopathic Structure

Whereas the schizoid withdraws, and the oral collapses, the psychopathic pretends. He imagines a better self and he attempts to manifest it in his appearance. The psychopath wards off the reality principle with imagination. As a child approaches the bridge of separation from the mother, the child must walk a path between dependence and autonomy. Separateness from the mother does not mean isolation, doing it alone. Rather, the separation that a child experiences as he or she crawls or walks away to explore represents a movement to relative dependence from absolute dependence, a balance of dependence and autonomy, a test of an intact sense of self. While the oral type stumbles back into extreme dependence, the psychopathic character veers off into an isolated, fantasized autonomy.

The psychopathic character has access to energy. Unlike the oral, the psychopath stood up and achieved a seeming autonomy

107

although at great cost. This character may have had to dig her mother out of the bar while quite young and wipe the puke off the floor by the TV where her father lay unconscious. This character type mothers and fathers the parents because often the parents were unfeeling caretakers or were narcissistically impaired themselves, incapable of loving others as separate individuals. The psychopath wins nurturing through premature adult behavior, including attention to appearance and image. Psychopaths' inner lives were not mirrored. They carry secrets never entrusted to others. Controlled through abuse and shame, they adopted their parents' manipulative power strategies rather than feel the terror of childhood vulnerability. Underneath the caretaking psychopathic structure is resentment at having been exploited and profound distrust in authority that they had to supplant on wobbly child legs. Pretending to be above need, they vicariously flirt with nurturing from a superior posture. Psychopaths pretend a strength they cannot sustain. They are restless and always hungry for something.

With this structure there is a propensity for domination and control, which is exercised sometimes with blatant disregard for others, shaming them. Others of this type, more subtle and thoughtful, manipulate people/situations to maintain distance and inner secrecy. Physically some members of this type are disproportionately developed in the upper body. They pull their energy upward, tightening at the diaphragm and failing to ground. They are always in flight. They do not dare to let down. Others have a beautifully proportioned body with a hyper-flexible back. They control more through seduction. The eyes of the psychopath are watchful and untrusting, although you may not know it. The type lives on charm, on magic. Figuratively speaking, no matter how rich they are, they live in their car.

Some very fine therapists have carried this structure, denying their own needs, eager to alleviate their loneliness by fanning the flames of gratitude in others. There is not enough love to fill the secret chambers of their heart. Some entertainers feel desperate between shows. No one penetrates to their secret isolation. They build walls of power and money to protect themselves from a vulnerability they dare not feel. They often present themselves for treatment only when everything has failed. Yet rarely will they admit their terrible pain. Instead they insist they are coming for "fine tuning" or as part of training or growth. They may try to humiliate and control the therapist after charming him, seducing him, or they may simply manage a safe distance and leave therapy when the distance is threatened by more than momentary closeness.

Within the same family is the narcissist. The narcissist identifies with his or her ego ideal. The ego ideal forms because the child, seeking to survive the loss of omnipotence, projects a sense of wholeness on to a parental figure. Later in childhood, he uses a friend or a superhero, a teacher or a ball player as his projected figure of wholeness. Through this projective identification one maintains an aspect of self intact and invulnerable. The developing ego can be resourceful at finding emotional support through desperate periods of childhood. What anguish a small boy suffers whose dad resents and ignores him. Even so he will make a hero of his dad against all evidence. He must find the admired object in order to go on, so weak and small, entirely at the mercy of an indifferent universe. A girl, emotionally abandoned by her mother, finds seductive attention from the father who misuses her trust. But the narcissist as a child finds no one around whose neck he can place this wreath of hope. These children could collapse in withdrawal and depression, but instead they take on the appearance of power. They place the wreath of hope, their ego ideal, around their own necks, a splendid ploy that keeps them in an imagined invulnerability. Untrusting of others and disregarding limitation, the intelligent and gifted narcissist can achieve great things in science, literature, art and politics.

The ego ideal is the forerunner of the super ego, the internalized parental voice. If we are not narcissistic, we may hold the ego ideal before us and feel the discrepancy between our present functioning and our perfect performance. We can tolerate both this discrepancy and the internal critic who speaks his mind. The narcissist, however, cannot tolerate the discrepancy and so denies it. When we deny the discrepancy between our real and ideal behavior, it becomes difficult to feel healthy guilt. Both the psychopathic and narcissistic characters feel above the limitations and ordinary rules of others since they experienced their parents as arbitrary and abusive, and therefore, dismissed their orders.

The psychopathic killer, the terrible extreme of this character, was something of a mystery to me until I read Melanie Klein's writings. She understood primitive rage and splitting, the lack of feeling and conscience before bonding takes place. I can imagine the semblance of adaptation without internal development or resource. We would like to take for granted the development of feeling and conscience as fundamental and a given in our humanity but we are foolish to assume that biology infallibly provides more than flesh and bone. Our full humanity is genetically a piece of good fortune and culturally and personally a hard won achievement.

When we talk with someone with a narcissistic defense, we begin to feel inadequate. we don't have a crease in our pants. Our dress feels suddenly frumpy. They, on the other hand, seem to be having a wonderful time. They are entertaining, full of energy and promise. They have no shadow, or they claim to have integrated it. We get to hold the shadow for both of us. They are the living fulfillment of their own ongoing dream and if their reality changes, they can adjust the dream. They are splendid sales people for themselves. In contrast, the psychopathic structure does not sustain a self myth with endurance and consistency. The shadow intrudes and is partially tolerated.

The narcissist cannot stand loss. Loss has been unbearable, and they refuse to experience it again. Their workers and their friends are all expendable. Their family must take comfort in their money and success, while they restlessly search for the inner food they have protected themselves against finding. Their inner life is secret and unavailable and often unknown and unreachable to themselves. If they betray their lovers, it has to be acceptable because they have always made their own rules. The psychopathic and narcissistic type have never let go of a childhood omnipotence. As a god or goddess you never have to have a bad day and the fault can always be out there with a tiresome, expendable humanity.

To work with the psychopathic and narcissistic structure, the therapist works to reach the secret self full of longing and need. We work to ground these structures, to move past bravado to feel the pain and weakness in the legs. The chest will most likely be frozen open, an inflated posture causing difficulty in expelling all the air in the exhalation. After gradual and gentle work, the client can use the barrel, the basketball or the stool to put pressure on the rigidly held chest. Eventually, the therapist works with the body-lying-down talking with the client to be sure that the posture is not too threatening. The purpose is to help the client let down, to suffer through fears of disintegration and allow support. In crisis, for instance with the loss of a lover, the underlying dependence of the character emerges in the face of denial. "I don't need anyone," he says but of course he does. Beneath the psychopath and the narcissist is the oral character he denies. Without the constant education, love and support of early childhood, the schizoid, the oral and the psychopath have no way to keep their balance in relationship, to be present, to maintain a balance between dependence and autonomy, and emerge with a functioning and durable sense of self.

The Masochistic Character

Roughly speaking, the transition from one and one half to two years old is a treacherous slide into limitation and cruel reality. At one and one half the child proudly has command. She stands confidently and runs and reaches. The child's pride at managing small tasks, and her busy language to herself speaks of an enviable world. With a loving mother or father near by, and joined with a god-like power, she has everything a child could want. But this world is precarious and short-lived, as her pleasure erodes into frustration. Perhaps it is the tree of good and evil children eat from as their consciousness brings forth separation and difference, and they come to test their will against the Lord of the Garden. How bitter and harsh the reduction, as the child, bereft, stumbles through the gates facing pain and smallness. The freedom of separateness is almost intolerable. No matter how loving the gods are, they cannot entirely cushion the fall from grace. During the developmental steps to follow, every gain is accompanied by severe loss.

The drama becomes unbearable when the parents are not accomplished and benevolent gods. If the mother cannot allow the child out of arm's reach because of her own desperate needs, how then can the child separate? If the mother cannot stand the child too close to her, how is the child to trust healthy dependence? Can a mother love a child more than her own life and then loosen her grip? For the psychopath, the self-absorbed parents needed him or her to serve them emotionally and sometimes sexually as the price for contact. Psychopaths never eat of the tree that might free them. They were never allowed to be small enough to distinguish good from evil. They stay in a bitter, desolate garden with the illusion of omnipotence to shield them against further growth. Everything looks right but the grass is astroturf and the flowers plastic. Often they have seen and experienced terrible things. How can they go on? There is no river to wash away grief, shame and memory. Such matters are buried deep in caves.

In contrast to the psychopath, the masochist has been attended to too well, not always with love, but with parental involvement. A parent is in the child's face and diapers all the time setting rules for right and wrong. In the anal phase, toilet training is carried out early with some harshness before muscular development supports the change. Feces, rather than being the precious product the child has made at the height of creativity, is smelly and disgusting. The child is shamed for not being clean. Spasms and contractions in the anal sphincter and pelvic floor, originating at this time may, in later years, interrupt genital function.

With a weary sigh, god drags the masochistic child out of the garden to a small shed where the child must stay to "think" about what he did. The psychopath refuses to acknowledge outwardly any shame, but the masochist is reduced to a more absolute obedience. Protest is crushed. If the child doesn't eat all the food on his plate, the father puts the food in the blender and makes him drink it.

The child sits at the table for four hours, until exhausted, she finishes dinner. She cries piteously. It is almost midnight and the tired parents are glad to go to bed. "Let that be a lesson for you. Your mother and father really do know what's best for you in every area of your life. Let us help you," they plead. The parents know what tastes good. The parents know what tastes good. And later on should the child want roller skates because her best friend got a pair and they are really cool, the parents rush out to buy the best pair and arrange for the best lessons, because the whole family were great on roller skates. The parents simply take over every idea, so that the child has no way to grow on its own. The parents can be well-meaning. "We don't think you should be friends with that boy." Their child will be smart and well dressed but can't finish papers. On the way to medical school, she has anxiety attacks at a key exam. She may manage a fine career but have no joy in it.

If the parents have good taste and judgement, perhaps every good thing has been spoiled for the child. The loss of her autonomy to the parent creates a terrible dilemma. If the masochist succeeds, she loses her soul because she is not fulfilling her own life but her parents'. If she fails, she has to live with a bad life. The masochist comes to therapy with hope and politeness. She flatters us and pushes us as therapists to perform. "I've heard good things about you. My last therapist was nice enough but nothing happened. He wasn't as bright, experienced and understanding as you. I've chosen you because I desperately need your help."

"Well," the therapist foolishly thinks, "What a nice person. I am good at what I do and I'm pleased my old client is saying good things about me out there. I'll be especially nice to this client. I'm lucky to be in the best profession in the world." Ten sessions later, the therapist and the client are painfully aware that absolutely nothing has happened. The therapist has never worked harder in her life. She has used every insight, every active process she has developed over years of trial and error. But the tension has grown thick between them. Clearly the client is enraged. She has been fooled again and has not paid for the last two sessions, and there is the hint in the air that she may not continue.

An oral client may enter therapy with hope and wonder and will experience disappointment and anger, but the masochistic client, in some cases sadistically humiliates the therapist in the ways he was humiliated and controlled by his parents. The rage and superiority underlying a veneer of civility falls heavy like a beating with a stick, and the therapist must wonder about his calling to this profession. With such a client it is critical in the beginning to place the responsibility of change with him or her. It is always important for the therapist to explore past therapeutic failures that clients report so that he can determine how this client defeats therapy. Otherwise he will be next in the trophy room where hang the sad heads of the weak who could not see through the character. Many masochists are genuinely seeking help and respect the truth. When the therapist lays out their dilemma, they are relieved and grateful. He tells them that he suspects they will be disappointed with him too, that they will in fact never get their therapists to change them. They are invested in defeating therapy, because the therapist becomes the parent invested in the outcome. If the therapist shows excitement in the least positive change by the client, the client will have to defeat the therapist by reverting to old behaviors once more.

The masochist complains. He holds great energy but cannot release it, much like a taut balloon unable to pop. In sadomasochistic practice, Reich felt that the masochist did not enjoy being beaten, but endured the pain because it triggered a release of tension otherwise not possible. The masochistic body tends to be short, thick and muscular, thick-necked, with the pelvis tucked forward. The masochist sits on unexpressed rage and a secret sense of superiority. Since the masochist endures and, thereby, loses feeling, the therapist works with kinesthetic awareness. Always one must uncover the secret resistance and make the masochist the ally or owner of the process. In grounding for vibration, does the client endure and resist a harsh direction by the authority, or does the client explore feeling for himself in his legs? There is some value to the therapist's pushing into the muscles of the neck and back but only if the client is actively engaged with him in "letting go."

The Rigid Character

The rigid character, having suffered in the Oedipal conflict, is proud and straight-backed with head held high, refusing to submit. He has survived the early childhood obstacle course and emerged as a winner with an intact sense of self. In Klein's terminology the rigid has attained the depressive position. The rigid has energy and direction, an aliveness that radiates from the core, and yet the rigid character holds back, afraid to be open. The rigid person felt rejected in his love affair with a parent and interpreted rejection of erotic love as rejection of love itself. Perhaps one parent prefers the child to the other parent and unconsciously is seductive while drawing back from the incestuous wish, creating a contradictory message that holds the child in bondage. The child retreats to an earlier developmental stage.

In this category we find the compulsive character, the phallic narcissist, and the hysteric, although these characters may appear more composites of earlier structures. The obsessive-compulsive character according to Freud fends off libidinal wishes and may reveal severe early damage covered over by an anal compulsive structure. The hysteric may be strong genitally or have a faint veneer of sexual play that overlays a schizoid or oral nature. Nevertheless, the attainment of the genital position, even with holding back, can be felt in the vitality and capacity for contact in most rigid characters.

In general when a child gradually separates from the mother, the child gives up imagined powers for the real, severely limited powers of a small being. Unable to understand the rules and purposes of the larger world, the child experiences constant, arbitrary interruptions in its efforts to explore and make sense of the environment. The child becomes a marauder, asserting its will in spite of interruption and disapproval. The child intensely feels its desires, needs, curiosities and angers, a proud child continuously in danger of the humiliation of being rendered powerless. Someone very large swoops down and scoops him up, like a hawk does a rabbit. At a moment of exaltation, the prized power object, the bread knife, is hurriedly wrested from his grip. He is left frustrated, amazed, hurt, humiliated.

If the child's caretaking has been predictable and kind, the child will be able to master its rage and bring the image of the good and bad parent into one constant figure, to whom trust can be extended even through the periods of insult. With what sadness a child must face the loss of magical ease and awaken to a raw external world that demands intelligence and discrimination. The child builds patterns of safety through higher functioning and pleasing the rule makers. The child builds power by flirting and achievement. The child smiles and the father melts. The child sits proudly in a little chair at a small table with a dish of cereal. He eats with a tiny spoon and the mother and father who created this small world for the child's benefit laugh happily as the child enjoys a sense of importance in a world that does not dwarf him.

No longer merged with the mother, separately sustained in dependence, the child's love affair individually with the mother and father excludes the other parent who ludicrously becomes the competitor. And the child whose head, heart and pelvis act as a single impulse does not understand the parents' reserve when the gestures are pelvically inspired. In the past, fear of castration and prohibition of masturbation was a credible explanation for injury at the Oedipal phase. However, today fewer parents threaten to chop off penises, and little girls are sometimes told that they are "fancy on the inside," in the words of Mr. Rogers. Nevertheless the breaking of the child,s pride, the humiliation of being treated as small, is often castration enough. The child with its tiny equipment cannot support an exclusive ownership of its beloved. In good-enough parenting the child is indulged and loved by the rejected parent rather than held to a competition. The child, loving both parents, runs back and forth, anxious and confused. Eventually the child must accept the loss of exclusive possession, and accept a further condition of being alone which prepares the way for best friends in pre-school and kindergarten.

At a younger age the child had to find a balance between dependence and autonomy in establishing a sense of self. At the Oedipal phase the child must walk between the Scylla of love and the Charibdis of aggression. If the mother is erotically attached to her son or the father drawn to the daughter as a younger wife, how is the child to escape being ground to pieces? Little boys have love affairs with their fathers and little girls with their mother. If unconsciously they are drawn in by a powerful tide, their small lives are in jeopardy. Rigid character results when the Oedipal conflict cannot be successfully negotiated. Drawn too close to the parent, the child must hold back, literally. The muscles tighten into the straightly held back.

For the rigid the early period of life was satisfactory for the development of an intact sense of self. The rigid is alive and well, competitive and in touch with reality. Her energy flows from the core to the periphery of the body. Muscular restriction does not inhibit achievement. The rigid knows he or she is loved and preferred. Sometimes it appears that the reality principle holds sway too much at the expense of pleasure. To win one parent in the Oedipal struggle binds the rigid character to an unconscious loyalty for life. Freud appears to have been a rigid character, who was very energetically alive, according to Reich. Freud's mother figured prominently in his life visiting every week for the many years of her long life. Freud was ambivalent about his father. He was extremely competitive and had difficulty letting people become close with him, unless he was clearly in control. He was as well heroic, generous and noble in thought. He was able to sustain himself through sudden impoverishment caused by the First World War, the loss of professional allies, the death of beloved family members, and painful operations for cancer of the jaw. As an old man he was courageous and defiant in the face of the Nazi threat and narrowly escaped with his family alive.

Energetically the rigid character holds in the long muscles of the body with spasticities in both the extensor and flexor muscles. The rigid character holds back trust and the heart, and turns therapy exercises into contests and performances to please the new parent. The Oedipal conflict must be revisited through a study of transference, personal history and body posture. What may prove most useful interpersonally is the study of the therapist's counter transference. The rigid's sexual nature must emerge in some form to be liberated and healed. Does the therapist feel pulled to respond seductively or to merge with the same sexed client, losing separateness? And how does the therapist respond to the competitive distance of the client? The rigid character can be far more difficult to work with than one might imagine, considering the absence of early damage. Often the rigid character is courteous and socialized and takes care of the therapist, a pleasant working relationship that may render the therapist powerless to intervene with ego dystonic insights. However, the body-lying-down and breathing provide a valuable access to the rigid client's full range of feeling without his having to engage the outer world. The therapist can disappear from view, since the client does not need reassurance, having an intact sense of self.

Chapter 16

The Family Body

> ... and a lonely man like yourself will perhaps find companions. But these companions are all in yourself, and the more you find outside the less you are sure of your own truth. Find them first in yourself, integrate the people in yourself. There are figures, existences, in your unconscious that will come to you, that will integrate in you, so that you may perhaps come into a condition in which you don't know yourself.
>
> C. G. Jung, *Nietzche's Zarathustra*

Some years ago, I ran a halfway house for people who had schizophrenic breakdowns. Many were young, in their twenties, and we fortunately put together a competent, loving staff. The family atmosphere helped clients come into a better balance with themselves. After some months working there, out of a clear blue sky, it occurred to me that I was working with schizophrenics, many of whom were considered chronic, and my oldest brother was schizophrenic. It had simply never occurred to me that there might be a connection. The mind may simply block out what it considers unpleasant and disconcerting.

I began at that moment to see myself as an extension of my family trying with what tools it had to resolve family dilemmas. I imagined a spider plant that sends out its shoots, which bend down and create their own roots, like children growing up and finding new soil. As children we unconsciously take on the unresolved

119

issues of our parents. We live out what remains unfulfilled in them. A mother who resents marriage because it aborted her academic career may have children who don't marry. A father who felt athletically inferior may find himself with children passionately involved in little league. Our children want us to be happy; they want to resolve our pain. They consider themselves at fault for our misery. At the very least they seek to stabilize us as parents so that they can have a safe environment to support their own growth.

Children must address the family's unresolved dilemmas as they grow to maturity or fall victim to the same problem. Children of alcoholics may overachieve to develop stability or collapse into the same disease. It is important that, as adults, we do not leave our lives unlived or our children may feel compelled to clean up after us. They will be driven to express what unconsciously we held in secret. Our children may never get around to living their own lives.

Not only are we left as children with our parents' unlived lives skulking in the shadows, their unresolved dilemmas, but we are unconsciously caught in their world view and their assumptions about every aspect of reality. We are caught in a subjective bubble, a projected, inherited universe a closed system, seeking solutions to problems that defeated our parents and using only the tools they have prescribed. If education is valued by a family member, then education becomes the over-determined source of answers. If money is valued, money becomes the solution. Rigidly doing the opposite of what we saw or was expected of us is of course, to be as deeply ensnared as our compliant siblings. Tragedy and severe conflict may be the only means to tear the envelope of inherited fantasy fashioned around us.

Even our bodies, having incorporated our parents' voice and gesture, are invaded. Is it only genetics that brings us to suffer from our parents' physical illnesses? We cringe when we see our father staring back at us in the mirror, the same halting bent shoulders and wry evasion. We adopt our mother's martyrdom, our father's despair as well as their appreciation for Bach and Mozart, their love of books. To deal with our father's body in ourselves is no easy task;

to differentiate ourselves from our parents is a complex analytic and a somatic task that calls for professional assistance. While we learn to accept our parents in ourselves, we identify our own gestures and our particular nature taking comfort in our separateness.

EXERCISE TWENTY: THE FAMILY MEMBERS

The client imitates his father. He walks like him, talks like him, gestures, sits down, gets up, whatever the client knows characterizes him. The client may need to start by talking about what it was like to sit at the dinner table with the father. The therapist may also enter the role-play as the father or the client. The client imitates other significant and impinging family members, the mother, uncles and aunts, brothers and sisters.

We carry other voices and bodies with us which we need to act out and identify. We take different forms which may not be identifiable as incorporated caretakers. We have subpersonalities we may come to know: the angry child, the vicious critic, the nurturing mother, the adventurer. We may find a voice and posture for them also. Such work is enhanced when pursued through an analytic bodywork.

One client introduced me to a very emotional and angry older man inside him who had his own history separate from my client's disciplined and rational personality. The rational Personality One wanted very much to see if I thought he was crazy. I drew no conclusions. I listened carefully to Personality Two and advised my client to do the same. The integration that took place was evidence of a personality structure flexible enough to be discontinuous and connected. In dreams we are often symbolically held in different forms. We are both the crazy man next door and the frightened neighbor. In conscious life we are likely to be alarmed or pathologize aspects of the self we have previously ignored or denied. We lose the flexibility of childhood when internal figures walk with us daily. Where I am not confronted with a blatant psychotic process in a client, I approach subpersonalities with respect and curiosity. They often further the goals of integration and internal balance.

Chapter 17

Shadow Body and Ideal Body

Everything on the planet casts a shadow. When an artist paints a dark side to an object, she makes the object look three dimensional. A shadow grounds us, gives us weight and credibility. Everything positive has a negative or dark side which we may accept or deny; in ourselves, the finest impulses have a dark brother, a Cain cast out, forever driven, a scapegoat, avenger, a monster hunting us in our dreams. And the body, which we cover so carefully, holds this shadow for us, the record of our denied selves kept from view like Dorian Gray's picture locked in a closet. The noble intellectual alternative, Dr. Jekyll, could not contain the physically brilliant, psychopathic Mr. Hyde. What we repress and deny comes upon us in time, biding its time through its locked expression in the body.

The body can only sustain a lie through character armor. The back of the body is often more shadowy, being less available to our own frequent inspection. Before a mirror we tamper with our front to look right. Our backside tells a blatant story of pallor, secret rage, poor diet, troubled childhood, depression and disguised collapse. Our posture reveals our bad attitude, our shadow body. Knowingly or unknowingly, we pantomime our unpleasant, denied nature which we thought we had left at home. If everyone learned to see the shadow body, I suppose we might integrate light and dark and become wise, or we might learn to hide our shadow in more obscure places. To look at the shadow body, we might first compare the back and front and mark the difference.

EXERCISE TWENTY-ONE: FRONT AND BACK

With your client standing observe his front and back, comparing the difference. Do both sides look like they belong to the same person? Is the front or the back built up? Is either underdeveloped? Does the spine seem to disappear and reappear? Does the front or back look all of one piece or in disjointed segments? Does the person look burdened, as if carrying a large weight? Observe from the side as well. Do any images come to mind? Take your time observing. Have your client close his eyes and become aware of what he feels in his body. So you can observe his back further, ask the client do a bend-over and, if appropriate to your stage of work, ask him to lift his shirt or use your hand to "see" more.

EXERCISE TWENTY-TWO: SHADOW BODY

In this exercise you want to note specifically, posturally, how your client stands in her darkened side. Imitate the posture to feel the positioning. How does your client's body organize itself to represent her shadow side? Ask the client to exaggerate the posture slightly so that she feels it. Often people slump and lock their knees. Their heads crane forward and their ankles collapse inward toward each other. They point their toes outward. Some people appear frightened, with their shoulders lifted and eyes averted. Others defiantly press the chest and chin forward while their legs are braced. If there is depression, how does it express itself? What is happening with your client while she stands in the slight exaggeration? When the position of your client is clearly identified and her posture described, move onto the next exercise, The Ideal Body.

EXERCISE TWENTY-THREE: THE IDEAL BODY

Ask your client to take an ideal posture. Perhaps she remembers a time when her body felt marvelous, a summer of swimming or hiking when she had time to relax and exercise. Imagining that time, your client takes her ideal body position and you record the stance, imitating the posture to understand the positioning of body elements. How does the posture feel to you? What are your counter transference responses? Ask your client how the posture feels to her. How hard is it to maintain the posture? Describe the posture to your client. For example, "You hold your shoulders back. Your back is straight and your chin is raised. You are looking off in the distance." Ask the client to talk about her associations with the "ideal" posture she has taken.

EXERCISE TWENTY-FOUR: THE SHIFT

When your client is clear about the elements that make up the ideal posture, have the client shift back to the shadow body. Ask the client how the shadow body posture feels now. What was the contrast in feeling between the two postures? Have your client switch back and forth between the two postures as if learning the movements of a dance. Take time with these exercises. Work with them over several sessions allowing opportunities to explore the emotional components of what is being revealed.

EXERCISE TWENTY-FIVE: A LADDER OUT

Having anchored both the shadow body and ideal body securely on a kinesthetic and conscious level, have the client make the transition from the shadow body to the ideal body in four movements so that, like rungs on a ladder, she has steps to take her out of the shadow signature. She may also reverse the steps so that she moves from the ideal to the shadow body. Clarify the emotional attitudes these intermediate postures represent.

The ideal body posture is probably not durable. It's often too extreme, too borrowed, too full of rigidity and perfection. Rather, we need to locate the liberated body, where posture expresses ease and strength. The ideal body denies the shadow, but the liberated body rests more in between, is more accepting of anger and sadness. The movements from shadow to ideal body help integrate ideal and shadow which forms the basis of our liberation.

EXERCISE TWENTY-SIX: THE LIBERATED BODY

Tell your client again to explore the steps of the ladder out of the shadow to the ideal. Modify and shift the steps if necessary, to discover a liberated posture in between the shadow and the ideal, a posture that is open but unstrained, that accepts the body's individual nature. We must not only give up the war with gravity through inner connectedness and balance, but also come to terms with superimposed ideals. A passion for physical perfection is often a desperate testimony to how unloved we feel. If we do not love and respect ourselves, we may place unrealistic demands on our appearance, to hide our deficiency. The body in recovery questions our cultural enslavement to stereotypes of beauty. Instead we turn within to feel our inner relatedness. We open to feelings and take pleasure in the ordinary activities of life.

Chapter 18

Eight Stations on the Journey up the Mountain

When I was young and built towers of blocks, I always built them in haste. Perhaps I was afraid my brother would knock them down before they were fully stacked. During those early days, I was more attentive to height than stability. In our haste to grow up, we are likely to settle for a stability which is uncertainly achieved.

In a process called "stacking," I have identified eight basic places where the "body blocks" join, where flexibility and stability vie for dominance. The eight stations are: the ankles, knees, leg/hip joints, lower back, mid-back and diaphragm, shoulders and arms, the base of the neck, and the occipital ridge (base of skull). The stacking of each block depends upon the balance achieved by the others. If our head cranes forward, it is futile to attempt to align it until the imbalances of the other junctures is replaced with greater flexibility. With restored mobility, the body reorganizes as it sees fit, in line with its innate sense of balance, energy, and well-being.

Stacking describes the price we pay for standing. If standing were not so difficult, perhaps we would find ourselves laughing in exultation at nature's triumphant ingenuity. Exuberantly we forgo the restrictions of crawling and lift up to a new world.

Standing up as children, our parents still tower over us. To stand like them frees our hands and arms to grasp what we want. We can move faster and see further. We are no longer just one piece. Now we have an upstairs and a downstairs, an upper and a lower body. Our coordination becomes more complex. Our pelvis turns and we must follow or our head turns and we must follow. What if our head and pelvis face in different directions? Are we divided by a twist? Like this can we go anywhere? And then one leg likes to lead. One leg likes to kick more than the other. One leg likes to go up the stairs more than the other and one arm and hand likes to throw the ball. These preferences may be faint or strong. They are routinely explored through repetitious movements until firm connections are made.

If being grounded in the world depends on our connectedness, then the eight key stations are essential for developing flexibility and relatedness. When we are undeveloped in our legs, arms or spine, key connections may be rigidly held or overextended in collapse. Exercises that explore a range of movement at the connection points, termed "stations," replace rigidity with flexibility and weakened structure with kinesthetic awareness and muscle tone. To feel the connection between our parts depends on repeated movements explored quietly and slowly with attention to pleasure and feeling. Small movements such as these engage the small musculature that is otherwise often overshadowed by large muscular movement.

There are people who have lost body function through accident and illness. They are likely to know a great deal about their injury and work repeatedly to regain partial use. But we who have lived all our lives with adequate functioning innocently disguise our injury through small compensations. Our bodies twist and bulge and stiffen in an effort to sustain our uneasy balance.

The eight stations help us feel our body's interconnectedness. If we are stiffly put together, how can we come into increased flexibility and better balance? Since we are learning to feel our body as it energetically awakens, we must give up our impatience and turn ourselves over to a meditative attention. To begin, we seek out our relatedness to our feet. Not merely doing exercises, we search out our nature and the nature of our feet. We wonder at the paleness of our ankles, the coldness of our toes. Images come to mind. We remember old injuries and feel the hurt we suffered years before, falling down the stairs. Women may remember shoes too small, forcing feet into "desirable" shapes. Sitting in a chair, we might turn our ankle reflectively, feeling the movement. We cannot be in a hurry to fix ourselves. We cannot expect explanations for every physical ache and structural anomaly, but we can hold our injuries in thoughtful reflection.

I talk of meditations up the mountain rather than mere exercises, because our task is ambitious. We shift our attitude and fundamental levels of our experience through unhurried attention. The exercises are presented as ways to develop interrelated structure and continuity of movement. So much depends on our willingness to evoke our body's withdrawn nature. We must not be in a hurry to change ourselves to match an ideal model that we deem correct. Instead we build a relationship to ourselves where we accept and love the ordinary, unnoticed experiences of embodiment.

It is enough to sit in a chair or take a walk. There is pleasure in reaching, turning or standing at the sink. If there is no pleasure in mundane movements, how can there be pleasure in anything? We live in awakened, felt experience and discover in small gestures the effortless form for our ongoing pleasure.

The First Station: Ankles

> Feet have to be on the ground, but I don't mean flat-footed. The bones of the legs have to be directly over the ankles. Now maybe you think that's a funny thing to say, but wait. In more than a quarter of the people you look at the weight does not go down across the ankle, through the middle of the leg. If you don't believe me, go and look. To be comfortable, weight must go through the middle of the joint, be it the hip joint, the knee joint, or the ankle joint.
>
> Ida Rolf, *Ida Rolf Talks*

Many exercises in grounding successfully bring movement and energy to this first connecting place, the ankle. Often we find energy blocked at the ankle as part of a larger standing complex. The ankle is rigidly fixed in partial collapse. The grey feet do not ground; the locked knees do not support. In these exercises, we interrupt the old pattern of muscular compromise and listen to the voices lost in frozen tissue.

EXERCISE TWENTY-SEVEN: GREY FOOT

Ask your client to massage his foot, to bring energy to it. The felt connection with the ground can then be explored. Direct your client to step barefoot onto a hard ball, and roll it into the arch and out, feeling the small movements of the many bones of his foot making adjustments. Have your client compare the feeling and coloring of his feet before working with the other. To confront his feet more intensely, the client may step on a broom handle, and starting with the toes, gradually inch his feet over it. His grey feet will flush with color.

EXERCISE TWENTY-EIGHT: ANKLE COLLAPSE

Standing with his weight primarily on one leg, your client works with his other leg, collapsing and straightening its ankle, rolling the ankle inward and out. After the client feels his range of collapse-straight, he settles somewhere near the midpoint of the ankle movement and lines up his knee directly with the ankle. Instruct him slowly to place some weight onto that leg. Your client repeats this exercise with the other leg.

EXERCISE TWENTY-NINE: ROTATING KNEES

This exercise promotes a wide range of ankle movement. Instruct your client to stand with her feet a few inches apart, parallel, and anchored to the floor. Bending her knees, your client rotates them in a circle. Although her feet are solid on the floor, she will notice ankle movement as she circles her knees.

The Second Station: Knees

A classic postural and energetic error is to lock our knees. We learn to lock our knees as an easy way to stand. When they bend back, we lean against the joint. As shock absorbers, knees need to bend slightly to provide play. With bent knees we feel our muscles flex and grow weary. We feel our legs supporting us, but often we prefer to feel nothing. With locked knees, we feel less, but the physical and psychic shock is absorbed by the lower back which becomes subject to injury.

EXERCISE THIRTY: STAND AND RELAX

Your client is to stand, bend her knees, and breathe. Encourage her to let her upper body relax allowing the lower body to provide her support.

This exercise can be practiced as you wait in line at the bank. Bend your knees and breathe. Sometimes, particularly at supermarkets, I like to feel the calves of my legs, particularly at supermarkets. Otherwise my legs just pass out like tired children. With bent knees, I go up and down on the balls of my feet, lifting the heel up and down until I feel the calves report in. "Hello down there." "Oh yes Sir, we're awake Sir." Knee rotation also is good for awakening energy.

EXERCISE THIRTY-ONE: THE CROSS CRAWL

Crawling can feel good if you have a soft rug and no knee injuries. As children we may have spent inadequate time crawling. We may have stood as soon as we could arrange it and missed valuable steps in coordination. In the cross crawl, we shift from moving the right and left side alternately to a more complex pattern where we move the right knee and the left hand, as a unit, followed by the left knee and right hand, a more advanced body circuitry than same-side crawling.

Direct your client to cross crawl. Be sure she alternates left knee, right hand, right knee, left hand and so on. If she has knee problems, have her check with her physician before working these exercises. Crawling on a mat, rather than the floor, can bring energy to the knee. Discuss the emotional impact of this exercise with your client.

EXERCISE THIRTY-TWO: KNEE SUPPORT

Typically as adults we no longer expect to be supported. We may carry in our stance a resentment for the loss of comfort and dependence. We may feel forced into adulthood before our childhood needs were met sufficiently. We may bitterly reflect in twilight flashes how unlikely it is that we will ever find support for who we are. Supporting the knees often releases deep holding in the client's body. Often the release is unthreatening and pleasurable and catches the client by surprise. The touching in this exercise can feel intimate and open us to deep feeling. Consider with your client whether the exercise is appropriate at this time.

Sitting on the floor, brace your back against a wall. Place your hands on your client's knees as they bend into you, accepting your support. For greater intensity look into your client's eyes. Discuss in detail the feelings experienced by the client.

The Third Station: Leg/Hip Joint

Many people contract at the ball and socket joint where the thigh joins the pelvis. The client is encouraged to stick his thumb into that socket and get acquainted with the tender or knotty tissue.

EXERCISE THIRTY-THREE: PULLING ONE'S LEG

While your client lies on her back, grasp her leg at the foot and ankle and, with her leg locked, gently push her leg into the socket. Then gently pull away and hold the position. As with all the exercises, the experienced therapist must decide whether an exercise is appropriate because of transference issues. Grabbing your client's leg may be entirely too sexual for you and some of your clients. If the exercise is not appropriate, light kicking, either lying down or standing up, is helpful. If standing, your client kicks as if she were tap dancing, a mere downward flick.

The Fourth Station: Lower Back

For many reasons injuries to the lower back are common. The lower back is often a place where rigidity is sustained, because we lock our pelvis into a position and inhibit feeling. If we lock our knees, the next critical juncture to absorb shock is the lower back. Perhaps we spend too many hours with our upper body tense and our pelvis glued to a chair at work. We need in our periodic work breaks to move our pelvis and back, to interrupt rigid holding.

EXERCISE THIRTY-FOUR: LETTING GO

Moving the pelvis with every breath, when we walk and even when we sit, is a natural and easy part of the body's innate pump of fluids and energy. Unfortunately, contrary to our body's organization, we tend to hold ourselves rigidly to avoid feeling in our pelvis. Perhaps we were once frightened by or warned against sexual feeling. Unable to release, we tend to push the pelvis forward or back.

Have the client swing the pelvis forward in a loose movement. Ideally the pelvis "lets go" as if dropping to swing forward. Ask your client to move his pelvis from side to side and in a circle. Work towards the client's flexibility and letting down for a natural sway when he breathes and walks. Let the client play with the possibilities of pelvic movement.

When the pelvis is rigidly held, ask the client to reach back to feel the back muscles attaching to the pelvis. Have the client place his hands on his lower back, the fingers pointing downward, the thumbs pointing outward. The client's hands are over muscles that may have lost feeling. To awaken feeling, he tightens the muscles cocking his pelvis back and up. After holding it for half a minute or so, he releases the area. Ask your client what he experiences. Is your client able to let go with the back muscles and let the pelvis "drop down"? Repeat until the client feels the muscles.

EXERCISE THIRTY-FIVE: BOUNCING

This is another way to loosen pelvic holding, The client, lying down, bounces the pelvis on a padded mat. Pay attention to your

133

client's breathing. Does she hold her breath? Does she hold her body in a rigid or relaxed way? What qualities characterize the entire body movement? After a few minutes, does the pelvis loosen? Have the client notices images and sensations during the bouncing process, to be discussed afterward.

EXERCISE THIRTY-SIX: FEELING THE LOWER BACK

Lying on her back with knees up and feet close together on the floor, your client gradually sways her knees from side to side, feeling the lower back through its movement. This exercise provides a safe way to explore feeling without stressing the lower back and also develops kinesthetic awareness. I found this exercise particularly useful for clients with back problems. The movement should be very slow, and when there has been injury, the range of motion should be limited, reflecting adequate caution.

The Fifth Station: Mid-back

What has been called an "oral collapse" describes the body caved in at the diaphragm, inhibiting breath. The mid-back responding to the collapsed chest forms a rigid arch. The oral collapse has been theoretically associated with difficulties in the first year of life concerning nursing and the lack or loss of mothering. The collapse may be quite subtle, inhibiting breath and restricting upper body movement.

EXERCISE THIRTY-SEVEN: ORAL COLLAPSE

To explore the midback station, The client collapses his chest as far as he can; and very slowly, attending to feeling, he extends and opens until he reaches the opposite position, that of extreme expansion. His back arches and his chest extends. Tell your client to move toward collapse once more. After he does a few cycles of gradual expansions and collapses, instruct your client to seek out a comfortable moderate position, one of openness he can maintain without undue strain.

Children are sometimes told to "sit up straight" by well-meaning adults. For that moment they adopt an exaggerated military stance with the shoulders pulled back, a posture that inevitably falls into collapse. The essential key to an open posture is feeling the spine and its support. Standing must be felt in the spine as well as legs. Our uprightness originates and is comfortably sustained through a connected spine.

EXERCISE THIRTY-EIGHT: BASKETBALL OR BLANKET

Have on hand a basketball or a tightly rolled blanket. Your client lies on her back on the floor, with the blanket or basketball under her mid-back. She can also explore other positions for the placement of the blanket and basketball which open her mid-back and diaphragm.

The Sixth Station: Shoulders, Arms

The shoulders lay upon the upper body like a shawl, attached at the clavicle (collar bone) while the scapula (shoulder blade) floats and slides on the upper back, loosely anchored by muscle. With difficulties in feeling the spine, and in an effort to stand straight, we often hike up the shoulders. The scapula ordinarily slides forward and back providing extraordinary motility and reach to the arms. With trauma the scapulae may anchor tightly to the ribs. The shoulders easily armor against life and lose motion. No longer do we reach out in tenderness or pull back to strike. The following exercises help release the unconscious holding.

EXERCISE THIRTY-NINE: SHOULDER LIFT

Ask your client slowly to lift her shoulders and hold them up tightly. This urges the contracted muscle to feel something other than its habitual holding pattern. Additionally, by exhausting the muscle, it may fully relax. After a few minutes, tell her to let go and let her shoulders fall. Repeat three or four times.

EXERCISE FORTY: CAT ARCH

The purpose of this exercise is to move the shoulder blades close enough to touch and as far away as possible in the reverse position.

On all fours, your client first arches his back and then reverses the arch. Touch your client's scapula as he arches and as he flexes into a reverse position. With your help, the client may feel his shoulder blades touch and slide apart.

EXERCISE FORTY-ONE: ARM VIBRATION

Your client is again on all fours, in an effort to establish vibration in the arms and shoulders. Your client does a few push-ups. It sometimes helps for her to have her hands and fingers point in toward each other. Remind her to keep her elbows unlocked. Once vibration is established, remind the client to breathe freely. Encourage her to sustain the vibration and see how far it extends through the body.

The Seventh Station: Base of Neck

The seventh juncture point is at the base of the neck. If the upper thoracic spine is flat and straight without its natural, gentle curve, the seventh station becomes the rigid platform that must support the neck and head. I have come to associate the scooped out, flat, empty quality of the upper back with emotional deprivation in childhood. Sometimes people develop mounds of flesh at this station, and their necks crane forward. When I was young, I found my hump very useful when I portaged canoes at a wilderness camp. Nobody else I know, however, has found the padding of flesh beneficial. Developing movement and energetic flow at the meeting place of the thoracic and cervical spine, the upper back and neck, depends on freeing up the rest of the spine below.

EXERCISE FORTY-TWO: UPPER BACK SUPPORT

Stand behind your client, and rest your hand at the base of your client's neck. After a few minutes, ask your client what emotions are present. Also place your other hand between your client's shoulder blades. Invite your client to lean back slightly into your hand while you provide support. Be sure you and your client breathe easily and freely. Some clients you may want to stand facing, offering support with your hand on the upper chest, so they lean slightly forward into your support.

EXERCISE FORTY-THREE: WEIGHTING THE HEAD

Ask your client to lock his hands behind his head, beginning a bend-over, and apply light pressure to feel his neck and spine. In particular, you want the client to regain feeling at the base of the cervical spine and the thoracic spine of the upper back. Working on the neck through massage is useful.

EXERCISE FORTY-FOUR: THE SWORD SWALLOWER

In this exercise, your client stands with his knees bent. You stand by his side and place a hand at the occipital ridge with the heel of this hand in back pushing against the spine as the head bends back. Your other hand at the forehead supports this movement. The client must maintain balance as his head bends backward. He feels the therapist's hand press against the upper spine. The client is asked to imagine he is swallowing a sword which must slip harmlessly down into the stomach. Encourage him to make a sound as if his voice reaches from the deep stomach area. Ideally his upper spine moves in the process. The exercise is useful in healing the oral collapse which depends also on regaining feeling awareness and flexibility in the upper spine.

The Eighth Station: Occipital Ridge

The top of the neck joins the skull at the occipital ridge, the last station, identified by Reich as the seat of blocking for what he called the ocular segment. This bony ridge of skull may be bunched with tight muscles. The neck muscles may contract tipping the skull backward and down. A row of acupressure points is located along the occipital ridge. even light touch here can relieve tensions.

EXERCISE FORTY-FIVE: THE MIRROR AND GOOSE

Have your client, in front of a mirror, explores what kind of movement is possible at this juncture. First, with her chin up, she extends her head and neck forward. Then your client reverses the movement, bringing her neck and head back in line with her spine. This forward and back movement imitates a goose. Then, ask her to drop her chin down to stretch the back of her neck. She repeats this sequence several times.

The eight stations for the body-standing-up join us as if we were nine blocks. They provide part of the answer to the issues of restructuring. We know that our flexibility is not a matter of freeing a few locations but the body as a whole. Nevertheless, the eight stations supply a necessary focus for exercises that interrupt the postural set of character. Enabling a greater choice in our movements, the exercises are easily strung together for a daily routine, or individually applied to the client's individual areas of difficulty.

It is through small steps that our body recovers. Gradually through incremental transformations of bodily attention, we sew the patches of consciousness together into a coat of many colors that is comfortable, elegant and simple.

Section Four

Protest and Emotional Expression

Chapter 19

Protest, Submission, and Surrender

My mother groan'd! my father wept.
Into the dangerous world I leapt:
Helpless, naked, piping loud:
Like a fiend hid in a cloud.
Struggling in my father's hands,
Striving against my swadling bands.
Bound and weary I thought best
To sulk upon my mother's breast.

William Blake, "Infant Sorrow"

At the heart of psychic injury is a crushed rebellion, a voice of protest reduced to silence. Without a voice, our broken spirit hates and despairs. We withdraw and deaden our feelings. Many people who outwardly submit will inwardly never surrender.

The husband, resenting the restriction, submits to marriage and deceives his wife. The wife, submitting to the wife-mother role, punishes her family indirectly. Outward passivity and inner secrecy poison our relationships. Consciously or unconsciously we sustain our rage and defiance under a cloak of smiles in a two-dimensional world, too frightened to express our true feeling. The capacity for grounded protest is a cornerstone of successful character analysis. There can be no acceptance of limitations, no full surrender of ego without first experiencing the unrestrained voice of protest.

Some dogs are yappy dogs. They protest as we approach the front door, but retreat fearfully, barking frantically, while other dogs, with a low growl, convince us to stand back. We must come to the low growl in ourselves to heal our brokenness. When, as children, we ascend the developmental stairs into our parents' larger world, we suffer progressive losses with each developmental gain. We lose the oneness with the mother and gain the freedom of separateness, but what a crushing loss of magical power and invulnerability! How small and powerless we feel. When our exclusive ownership of the mother is challenged, our young hearts are broken, and yet we gain the father's comfortable authority. We are fortunate indeed if our genes give us adequate raw material and if there is a good match between our needs and our family's capacity to give. If our parents guide us firmly, mirror us lovingly and love each other, we will tolerate the limitations which cruelly push back our narcissistic expectations. We may even flourish. If on the other hand we have extraordinary needs, or our wounded parents fail us, we may hold all authority in contempt and refuse to bow down to the restrictions of ordinary life. We may consider ourselves special, exempt from life's tedium. Enraged or compliant, we deny and oversimplify reality, failing to integrate new experience.

We are easily frightened as children. Eating what we hate, kissing those we distrust, we act to win approval. Verbal and physical abuse leave us blaming ourselves with no way to gather sufficient self to protest. Our character is evidence of our accommodation to a world that denied us honest expression. In an analytic bodywork, we must protest at the site where our submission was demanded. If we swallowed down foods and opinions we hated, we may have to vomit them up. If we bore childhood burdens on our bent back, we may have to throw off the burden repeatedly. If our arms dared not reach out to protect us from abusive verbal and physical blows, we may need to push and hit. If we were sexually violated, we may need to struggle and kick to feel power protecting our lower body from unwanted intrusion. If our mouths and throats were invaded, we may have to cough, spit, shout, bite, growl and push away. Our understandable failure to protest as mistreated children to avoid further pain, nevertheless, feels like cowardice to us, a cowardice we repeat through small avoidances of conflict.

142

We hide our protest through control, collapse, displacement of affect and acting out. Controlled people become impenetrable and distant. No one, they hope, will be able to humiliate them again. Others tighten their jaw, biting down against rage and disappointment, contracting the chest and shoulders to hold back expressions of pain and violence. In collapse some people give themselves over to anxiety. Through submission they hope to avoid further pain. They say to the persecuting inner voices, "I'm ill. You can't punish me now." Or they say, "See what pain I'm in. It's your fault." Often in collapse the rage shines through as blame.

Some people split off from negative feelings. They become indifferent to abuse. Their rage transfers to a safer target or remains split off and lost. In the psyche, feelings appear to be set adrift in an ocean where they might never be found, but the body teaches us that no persistent feeling is ever lost. Its path is meticulously recorded in flaccid or contracted tissue. No split off feeling escapes the body's net of tissue. By acting out some people find momentary protection from fear through explosive rage. Others behave with reckless abandon adopting a fearless manner as if they have nothing to lose.

The forced submission of rape exacts a terrible price in traumatic injury, but may not silence our protest. Submission is the stopgap measure we take when we are afraid and overwhelmed. We would not fully submit to physical, verbal or sexual abuse if we could gather ourselves in protest. If we could call forth a sufficient sense of self, at least we would sustain our protest secretly. As a desperate withdrawal, submission contradicts the five principles of contact. Submission disconnects us from our ground, painfully demonstrates our violated boundaries, cuts us off from feeling, restricts breathing and erodes our intention. The substrata of submission is ungrounded rage. Hence, all bodywork that disrupts body armor and establishes contact, i.e., the body in recovery, evokes our hidden protest.

If our literature is a measure, in the nineteenth century, people still believed in the power of the will to fend off seduction, violence, betrayal and fear. Men and women of courage could endure anything until, in the twentieth century, our unconscious desires compromised our heroic purity. Certainly male vanity lost its flawless erection in recent wars, faced with advanced techniques of brainwashing. When the terrorized Patty Hearst was allowed out of the closet, she helped to rob a bank with her abductors. It appears that everyone can be broken with sleeplessness, abuse, and drugs.

In her brilliant book, *Trauma and Recovery,* Judith Herman compares victims of sexual and domestic violence to survivors of military combat. Encountering a rapist, "The women who remained calm, used many active strategies, and fought to the best of their ability were not only more likely to be successful in thwarting the rape attempt but also less likely to suffer severe distress symptoms even if their efforts ultimately failed."[1] A study of ten Vietnam veterans who survived heavy combat without post-traumatic stress disorder, reveals men who stayed calm, retaining good judgement, who stayed in contact with others and preserved their moral values and sense of meaning. They were characterized by a "triad of active, task-oriented coping strategies, strong sociability, and internal locus of control."[2] While all of us can be broken, there are qualities of self that best assure our survival.

Self has no permanence. Self is a construct programmed in childhood. To protest we need a stable, related self, with a continuing emotional reference that builds memory, a point of view, and a consistent strategy for living. Self as a construct rather than an immutable given, must be sustained in the same the way a fire must be fed. People brought up with a damaged sense of self often resent having to sustain themselves through disciplined effort.

My laptop computer has no fixed memory. If I leave it untouched in its case for a week, the programs are lost. Its hardware, however, retains its inherent capacities. If adequately maintained, my laptop operates as if it had a hard drive and fixed memory. Similarly, our bodies retain our instinctual organization capable of primitive functioning, but our sense of self calls for high maintenance and high definition. With sufficient attention, our self construct can be a solid wall to put our back against.

Children from "good" families develop a solid sense of self, an identity they can count on which seems as permanent as the body itself. They are told as babies that they are cute, wanted, wonderful, loved, smart, and very special thousands of times at all hours of the day and night. They are listened to, heard and respected as separate individuals and encouraged to develop their own interests and opinions. They are capable of protest and do, but are also firmly directed by parents they can trust and respect. The countless hours of training the self received in such families cannot be made up for in later years by a few affirmations and words of encouragement.

Building a functional and durable self is a central task of therapy. Our self construct takes shape through countless varied interventions. We develop stability insofar as we are able to integrate the shadow in our lives. If we idealize or devalue, and split off and project the good and evil parts of ourselves on to others, we will remain profoundly confused about who we are. As well. many people stabilize themselves by borrowing a group identity. The passionate affiliation to the old school, a sports team, a profession, their country, may be partly fueled by a shaky sense of self. And when the ego reduces life to bite size because everything new is a threat, the great archetypal experiences of birth, love, death, beauty and terror that connects us to humankind throughout the ages, is denied. For good reason, we must war against the trivializing of our lives. When we ground, when we establish good boundaries, open our breathing and access our feeling, we establish a functional and durable self where protest and surrender are possible.

With the self intact, and protest an option, surrender now becomes possible. Surrender is a supreme act of self very different from submission. Surrender is the ability to let go, to accept what is going on rather than hold to an imagined life, the way we think our lives ought to be. Our surrender can be purposeful and intended as well as a spontaneous response to a life event we are ready for. "Of course," says Jung, "the indispensable condition is that you have an archetypal experience and to have that means that you have surrendered to life."[3] When we surrender in sexual intercourse or to a Higher Power, the giving over of willful control is a remarkable and profound act, not possible without integrating the rage beneath our submission and grounding our protest, so that we are in contact with ourselves and others.

Chapter 20

Emotional Expression

> A purely disembodied human emotion is a nonentity. I do
> not say that it is a contradiction in the nature of things, or
> that pure spirits are necessarily condemned to cold intellec-
> tual lives; but I say that for us, emotion dissociated from all
> bodily feeling is inconceivable.
>
> William James, *The Principles of Psychology*

While human nature produces a bewildering combination of possibilities, geniuses, idiots and a range of originals in between, there
remains only a small number of key aspects to our make-up. Our
emotional life shares preeminence with intelligence, imagination,
creativity, humor, physical prowess, beauty, qualities of character,
wisdom and spirituality. People who lack in one quality compensate for it by strength in other qualities, but when they lack feeling, the very nature of their human experience is threatened. In
criminal cases we are most appalled by the offenders' absence of
feeling. Although we are shocked by the terrible things people do
to others, the deficits of feeling face us with a humanity that is
monstrous, that we consider inhuman.

Feeling is not only instinctual but also develops through mod-
eling, correction, nurturing and attention. Dysfunctional families
teach us to disregard the complexity of our feelings and rob us of
precious years of positive learning. We often emerge as adults unso-
cialized, ego-centric and inappropriate in our behavior. Sometimes

we are split off from feeling and sometimes our feeling is primitive. Both conditions make contact impossible.

Theorists differ as to how injury to feeling comes about, whether primarily in an interpersonal or intrapsychic manner. Wilhelm Reich considered the infant as open, emotionally present, demanding and aggressive in a naturally healthy way until such time the child's needs are unmet by adults. The child defensively turns against itself, inhibiting expression, creating a split between core feeling and an adaptive face. An unhealthy, sexually repressive culture perverts innately healthy nature. This view of man, an interpersonal model, is constructed from the early Freudian model of instinctual repression.

On the other hand, Melanie Klein, adapting Freud's intrapsychic model of drives, saw the infant faced with internal conflicts of feeling from birth, love emanating from an instinctual drive drawn toward life, while hate, destructiveness and envy proceeded from the death instinct. The infant does not perceive the mother as a whole person at first but relates to the breast as an object. The child is soon faced with the "good" breast that nurtures and the "bad" breast that fails to fulfill its needs. When the mother does not respond immediately to the child's need, the child feels rage toward what becomes the "bad" breast and projects its rage onto the bad breast which it fears will retaliate violently. The bad breast as persecutor arouses intense anxiety in the child and so the child must split it off to protect the integrity of the good breast. The child incorporates the good and bad breast which become internal representations in the child's mind. The persecuting bad breast becomes the foundation of the super-ego or child's conscience. Only later is a child able to perceive the mother as a whole being rather than "part objects."

Hence the splitting of feeling is the inevitable first step in life. Good parenting promotes feelings, allowing access to their full range. The child feels sufficiently safe in the family that she can accept frightening thoughts and feelings which might otherwise overwhelm her young consciousness. The splitting off of "bad" feeling, however accomplished, leaves us diminished in our humanity in ways that disrupt our capacity for intimacy, contact and pleasure. If we have pain in our foot and we numb out the pain, functionally we have only one foot. In the long run, we need both feet even with the pain. Our feeling gives us the sense of being present in the room here and now. From such inclusive feeling comes the manifestation of body awareness.

It has always been easier for mankind to project the shadow onto the enemy, to find the darker range of feelings abundantly in evidence in our husband, wife or child but fail to see the same qualities in ourselves. It is easier to be unreasonably frightened of spiders than to search out the internal, split off feelings of primitive terror in ourselves. When we project our blind side onto others, it may be the only way we can contact that lost aspect of our being. Projection, more than a mistake, may become a tool to observe ourselves, a step in self-discovery.

How do we gain access to our emotions? Often the underlying feeling jumps out at us when we exaggerate postural states. Introducing movement to rigid structure can kick loose hidden feelings. Through gentle inward attention and kinesthetic awareness, feeling can be experienced. Reich felt that inhibiting respiration was the primary neurotic mechanism to repress emotion: breathing fully into our chest and belly releases emotion.

Overview of Reich's Work

As a young doctor and a member of the Vienna Psychoanalytic Society in the early 1920s, Reich developed a theory that all neurosis was caused by somatic conflict through the damming up of libidinal energy. Psychic conflict without biological support could not cause neurosis. Reich extended Freud's concept of actual neurosis to include psychoneurosis. Reich felt that developmentally, libidinal energy dammed up through repression at the oral and anal stages and then was not available for genital release. The repressed sexual energy was experienced as anxiety in the respiratory and cardiac systems where typically it located itself, although anxiety might transfer to other areas like the intestines. Energetic disturbance in the heart area awakened mortal fears and secondarily took on psychological meaning. However, Reich's work to release dammed up sexual energy at pre-genital fixation points did not consistently establish genital function. If dammed up energy was not being held entirely at pre-genital hideouts, where was the energy held hostage? Anxiety, the dark twin of sexual pleasure, Reich discovered, was also bound by character, the entire body attitude.

Psychoanalytic practitioners who opposed Reich's genital theory argued that they had neurotic patients who had healthy sexual lives. They bragged of male sexual athletes who "came" many times in one night. After some reflection, Reich argued that such behavior was evidence of a failure to surrender in a full release, and that the clients might have pre-genital fantasies of the penis as a piercing instrument. Excessive erectile potency might mask a fear of women and serve as a defense against homosexual fantasies.

As a result of this challenge, Reich formulated a concept of the sexual embrace that called for the surrender to the biological process. In the orgasm process, Reich initially observed how different body systems were engaged. At first sexual energy accumulates in the vegetative system without tension. During the sexual act excitation concentrates in the genitals. Pleasure gathers throughout the sensory nervous system to a climax, release comes through the motor nervous system and musculature. With the release of tension, a feeling of pleasure pervades the whole body.

Reich came to understand the body as a longitudinal bladder with organs and tissues of different densities conducting bioelectrical charges through the length and breadth of the organism. Energy was dispersed from areas of greater to areas of lesser charge, but consistently through-out, from the center, where energetic charge generates, to the periphery. Unobstructed, the building and releasing of charge creates rhythmic expansion and contraction, a pulsation natural to all living organisms. Through expansion the organism increases tension while the discharge releases tension.

In particular Reich noted a four beat process whereby an organism swelled and contracted which he called the "orgasm formula."

He noted that in sexual interchange, mere mechanical swelling was not sufficient for a person's pleasurable sense of release but that tumescence must be accompanied with electrical charge for a person to experience the discharge as complete and pleasurable. Hence, the orgasm formula distinguishes between electrical charge and mechanical swelling: mechanical tension, electrical charge, electrical discharge and mechanical relaxation. Through experiments in the 1930s, Reich established that bioelectrical energy, generated in all living organisms, was the source of pleasure in the pulsation process and a tangible identification of Freud's libido concept. The orgasm reflex was the prototype of all pulsation in its energetic buildup and release, a universal biological reality that shared its central importance only with the pulsation of breathing. With the development of vegetotherapy in 1934, Reich was able to address the psyche-soma relationship directly.

Reich's bodywork, always biologically based, became increasingly independent of depth psychology and verbal therapy. With his discovery of the cosmic orgone energy, Reich had the unifying concept that dissolved the distinction between psyche and soma. Orgone therapy works with the expansions and contractions of plasmatic currents with the "holding back" in the organism. "We have left the realm of psychology, including 'depth psychology,' and have even gone beyond the physiology of nerves and muscles into the realm of the protoplasmatic functions."[1]

"Basically, emotion is an expressive plasmatic motion."[2] Emotion, Reich said, literally means "moving out" which describes the expanding plasmatic motion of pleasure. The plasmatic motion from periphery to center is experienced as anxiety. When the patient comes with problems, the therapist need not listen long to the words, but instead observe their expressive movements and emotional expression. Reich felt that the expressive biological language of the core being was far beyond the reach of words. To work, therefore, at the core level requires a silence, a stillness of observation that calls forth the life force to free itself from its inhibitions. The orgone therapist holds the client as a whole being, no longer supporting a defensive split between psyche and soma. To Reich it was more important to work with the expressive language than with individual muscles.

The body may be seen in a simplified and humbled form as a worm or snake that unimpeded, ripples with energy. Yet what happens to the organic wave-like motion, speculates Reich, if any portion of the snake is tied down? In just such a manner we experience character armor. The muscular armoring prevents the orgasm reflex from occurring. The orgasm reflex is that wave of excitation like the rhythmic movement of a snake that runs from the vegetative center in the pelvis throughout the body over head, neck, chest, abdomen and legs. Reich worked to established the orgasm reflex in his clients. Reich saw the body as split into seven segments when its pulsation was interrupted, seven rings at right angles to the flowing current: the ocular segment, the oral segment the cervical, the thoracic, the diaphragmatic, the abdominal and the pelvic segment. Because Reich worked with people lying down, he felt that release of armor should take place proceeding from the head toward the pelvis. If energy were released in the pelvis before armor dissolved in the head and chest, the damming up of energy might prove unpleasant and dangerous.

Reich's work promised to clear the person's physical barriers to natural, energetic flow. The promise was to release the body's energy fully through the orgasm reflex, to allow the body once more to clear itself periodically of tension, for the body fluids to well up and release without blockage and stagnation. Reich's system also promised to reach directly down into the unconscious life to release all trauma, all memories that held back the emotional flow of life, to release the split off feelings so that they returned to the body's emotional totality. Reich felt that Freud's free association method aimed for the unconscious but grasped at derivatives, while his own method of orgone therapy moved directly to free the instinctual life.

While some critics feel that Reich made extravagant claims, his methods have continued to successfully release deep levels of feeling, and opened up memories not otherwise accessible through traditional psychotherapy. Derivatives of Reich's work in which lying down and breathing deeply are major components are to this day winning converts, despite such a cathartic method remaining revolutionary and frightening to outsiders. Lying down and breathing deeply for an extended period of time, one to two hours for instance, accesses feeling and lost memories. Lying down, a person tends to regress, to act and feel much younger, to feel basic emotions more intensely, to bypass defensive armor. These kinds of techniques are valuable when directed by competent professionals trained in the work; we do not want our clients' unconscious to unleash more than they can handle at one time. To access the full range of emotional expression so intimately knitted in somatic fabric, we can follow the genius of Wilhelm Reich in his vegetotherapeutic work.

Chapter 21

Hitting

The spotted hawk swoops by and accuses me,
he complains of my gab and my loitering.
I too am not a bit tamed, I too am untranslatable,
I sound my barbaric yawp over the roofs of the world.
                    Walt Whitman, "Song of Myself"

As children we were often powerless to defend ourselves against the force of our parents. By nature we hit and kicked, but such actions may have been ruthlessly suppressed as shameful and ungrateful expressions. We had to go to school and be silent. We were trained to be docile in a restrictive world. The world applauded our servility provided we were not too obvious about it. Sooner or later, however, we are visited by the deep winds of despair since a life of submission has taken from us our most prized creative nature and turned us into foolish reflections of other people's imagined wishes. If I paint too dark a picture, I fleetingly take refuge in the moral tradition of Thoreau who stated that most men live lives of quiet desperation.

As infants we turned away from our mother's breast when she was late in returning. We refused to look her in the eyes. Sometimes we protested by arching our back or kicking. Later we protested by lying down, by kicking and screaming and "getting out of control." Sometimes such protests drove our parents mad with rage and they beat us with words, fists or belts and we cowered before the giants' greater force of madness.

But some of us had parents who were able to understand our protests, help us to contain ourselves and firmly lead us into reluctant cooperation. We could trust them sufficiently to accept their parental authority, and dimly we understood that they had our best interests in mind. Those parents instilled in us the belief that we could negotiate or cooperate with authority without sacrificing something essential in ourselves.

Our socialization demands of us the containment of aggression. In our rush for approval, we may split off hostile feelings, living with little awareness of our shadow. We lose access to a great range of feelings and live in emotional poverty. Instead of being direct, our anger seeps out in convoluted or twisted ways.

Exercises in hitting and kicking provide the opportunity to become kinesthetically and psychologically aware of repressed aggression. With effort we may open up feelings tied up in tissue, lost to unconsciousness. We may integrate split off feelings as we exercise our body in recovery. Because it helps the client feel active, protected and empowered while opening to deeper feeling, I have used hitting early in the therapy process. But some people are afraid to express anger in my office. They think they are unleashing a curse. They do not realize that it is hidden anger that curses them every day. What is unexpressed is perfectly preserved, unable to resolve or release. Hitting and kicking clears the feeling by bringing it into the light of day. If your client should, however, experience some fear or vulnerability that feels uncomfortable, then stop the exercise and talk about the experience.

EXERCISE FORTY-SIX: THE HITTING MEDITATION

In my office I have a fat plastic bat purchased at a toy store for three dollars. The bat, swung overhead and down against a foam cube, makes lots of noise and is most pleasing to hear. Some people use a tennis racket against a pillow, bed, or couch. Also, hitting can be safely done with the whole forearm; using only the fists, a person can hurt his or her wrist through its bending.

Hitting against a foam cube or bed, the client stands, but to hit a low pillow, the client kneels or sits. Direct your client to hit the cube or pillow and to pay attention to how the body feels. The point is not to hit hard to impress others, but to focus on inner attention. Encourage your client to feel the relatedness of body structure or its lack of connectedness. The client may feel the energy as it gathers and shifts or an awakening desire to hit harder.

As the client hits, have her observe what "inner movies" are playing, what images become conscious. Sometimes the faces of people appear. Sometimes the client remembers an earlier conversation, the emotional content finally declaring itself. In the hitting meditation we begin to clear the body-psyche of debris collected over years.

EXERCISE FORTY-SEVEN: WORDS AND PHRASES

In this exercise the client uses words and phrases to direct his attention. The client hits and says "no" for ten hits, then "I won't," followed by "Stay away." Encourage your client to use a vulgar expression or two if he wants to find phrases that are his own. Both you and your client notice which phrases awaken the most energy. Remind the client, as he hits, to bend his knees and feel his legs. If hitting ungrounds him, he may need to slow down. Have him breathe into his lower belly. Lead him to grounding exercises before he resumes hitting.

EXERCISE FORTY-EIGHT: TANTRUM

Your client lies down on her back on a foam mat. Tell her to hit it lightly at first to warm up. After a while, tell your client to extend her arms over her head for a full swing, and as she hits the mat, she turns her head from side to side. And now, including her legs, the client kicks with full effort. You want to be sure that when the client lets loose with a hitting and kicking tantrum, she does not injure herself by hitting or kicking nearby furniture.

The tantrum has the possibility of a cathartic release. Its often more effective to encourage your client to "give all you've got" for a short period, rather than make a longer less vigorous effort.

EXERCISE FORTY-NINE: ELBOW HITTING

Once again on her back, lying down, your client hits the foam mat, but this time she uses her elbows. Let her elbow hit with her arms by her side and also away from her body. Try the same exercise with the client standing backed up against a foam pad leaning against the wall. This exercise helps bring movement and feeling to the shoulders and shoulder blades, and brings up resentments and angers otherwise lost.

EXERCISE FIFTY: KARATE HIT

Standing with knees bent, the client makes tight fists and brings both her elbows back. To make a fist, the client stands with palms up and slowly curls her fingers toward her palm. She keeps her thumb on the outside curling it tightly across the knuckles just above the nails. If your client were to open her fists now, the palms would face upward. To throw a punch, your client brings her fist forward while turning it. When her fist hits, the twist has brought her palm to face downward. Ask your client to alternate hitting with each arm, exhaling with each punch.

EXERCISE FIFTY-ONE: KARATE ELBOW

Ask your client to stand with knees bent, elbows back and fists at waist level by his sides. Instead of bringing his fist forward, he brings the elbow forward to strike. In bringing his elbow forward, his fist curves across his chest. Tell your client to alternate blows from each elbow. The elbow hit helps to loosen the shoulders.

Chapter 22

Kicking

He clasps the crag with crooked hands;
Close to the sun in lonely lands,
Ring'd with the asure world, he stands.
The wrinkled sea beneath him crawls;
He watches from his mountain walls,
And like a thunderbolt he falls.

Alfred, Lord Tennyson, "The Eagle"

Our aggression may fall upon us from the heights or rise from the depths. We must not blame our "lower" selves for our aggressive nature. We are more complex than that. Nevertheless, the lower body that supports us is metaphorically associated with our earthy, instinctual animal nature whose power is represented by the centaur rather than the eagle. We may also associate our efforts at integration with Hermes, messenger of the gods, the "patron saint" of robbers whom travellers appealed to for protection. Hermes moved easily between darkness and light, the realms of heaven, earth, and underworld. He was a god able to integrate the shadow of our lower nature in its violence, longing and lust with higher expressions of power, spiritual awareness and generosity. Within our pelvis is the key to connecting our dark and light selves. The unconscious finds its first home in the lower chakras. Held in the deep waters of the pelvis, it may rise up to cloud every aspect of body. Our life energy, the kundalini, like the fiery sun rising out of the ocean, moves above the surface of the earth—marked in the body by the diaphragm—on its heavenly journey through the upper body and into the higher realms of air, intellect and spirit.

Locked within the pelvis resides years of unexpressed feeling, sometimes angry protest, passion, longing, memories of incestuous assault. Kicking, natural to a centaur, unlocks the feeling power of the lower body, connecting the feet, legs and pelvis, and opens an energetic path to the belly and upper body. In this way, kicking addresses the deep split between the upper and lower body. Darker sexual memories may emerge with sustained kicking. Sometimes people experience more pent-up energy in their lower than upper body. The client can find pleasure and release in kicking.

The following exercises allow you and your client to explore a range of emotional expressions. As a body therapist, you will want to do these essential exercises yourself to help you maintain contact with unconscious emotion. Notice whether kicking grounds you, excites you, releases you, energizes you, angers, frightens or saddens you.

EXERCISE FIFTY-TWO: KICKING LYING DOWN

On a comfortable futon or mat, the client lies down on her back and kicks a few times. With legs loose and moderately straight, she alternately lifts her legs and then kicks them downward, like a scissors. Direct your client to explore kicking lying on her belly as well. Sometimes it is useful for the client to kick in short bursts with great intensity. If the client is lying on a hard surface like a floor, with knees up, she stamps. The emphasis is on the gesture rather than harsh contact. While your client kicks, remind her to be in touch with, and to report, images and feelings/emotions that surface.

EXERCISE FIFTY-THREE: STANDING KICKS

Brace a foam cube against your knees and ask your client to kick it standing, making contact with the ball of the foot rather than toes. Words may arise. One client spontaneously began saying,

"Get out of the way," as he kicked. Tell your client to stay aware of his feelings as he kicks; feelings are often identified with specific gestures. At home, without your assistance, a client may try to kick a cardboard box propped against the wall or a large pillow or a futon folded and propped up.

EXERCISE FIFTY-FOUR: STAMPING

Some animals stamp in warning. Stamping touches in to early childhood gestures of anger and protest. While standing, the client stamps with intensity for a brief time. Your client also may stamp with moderate emphasis for a few minutes. Perhaps words will come to mind that the client says like "That's mine," "Listen to me," or "I won't."

Chapter 23

The Ocular Segment—Uncovering Feeling and Protest in the Eyes

Anxiety may be compared with dizziness. He whose eye happens to look down into the yawning abyss becomes dizzy. But what is the reason for this? It is just as much in his own eye as in the abyss, for suppose he had not looked down.

Sören Kierkegaard, *The Concept of Anxiety*

I would like to think that I see what others do not see and that years of experience have paid off in heightened sensibility, but I have found that when I point out seemingly subtle qualities of light and energy on the body to trainees, they see them too. As beginners, however, they hadn't looked for this or didn't have a vocabulary to differentiate one energy state from another.

The eyes, for instance, provide a remarkable range of identifiable expressions which are easily described once we give ourselves permission to do so. Children may develop boundaries in their eyes, blank stares that let no one in. Those same eyes acting as interior walls, may be flashing with intelligence, sex or humor. Soft, tender, bright or hard as marbles, the eyes remain impenetrable. Other eyes invite us in. We see the subtle interplay of feeling as it takes place in them. We are brought into the home rather then left standing outside like an untrustworthy salesman. Many people search outside themselves for clues about their safety. Working hard to observe, They do not think the light will come to them, that they may relax and bring images from the outer world into the comfort of their inner world. So much can be read in the eyes: anxiety, compassion, tenderness, sexual feeling, playfulness, serenity, coldness, lassitude, distance, ill health, anger, contempt, despair, and even death.

The ocular segment includes hearing and smell. The muscles of this segment, including those of the eyeball, eyelids, the forehead, tear glands, flesh on either side of the nose, the deep muscles at the base of the occiput, and even the brain are involved in contraction especially with shock and withdrawal. People who were party to frequent family fights may not want to see, having established characterologically a selective blindness. They may not be able to cry.

EXERCISE FIFTY-FIVE: NAMING

Look into your client's eyes for a while. Vary the distance between you. Do you see fear? Are you allowed inside or kept coolly at a distance? Do both her eyes seem the same? Share your observations describing the feelings, the movements and shifts you observe in your client's eyes.

EXERCISE FIFTY-SIX: MIRROR

Bring your client to a mirror, one on the wall or a hand mirror. He looks into a mirror at his eyes. Can he let himself in? Tell him to relate what he observes? Does he see both his eyes as the same or different?

EXERCISE FIFTY-SEVEN: THE LIGHT COMES TO YOU

Have the client close her eyes and gradually open them, letting the light of the room come to her. Tell her not to effort to see, but to let the images come to her and form on her retinal screen in the back of her eye.

EXERCISE FIFTY-EIGHT: PUSHING CHIN

Your client lies down comfortably on his back with his head on a pillow. Sit to one side of him by his chest and apply mild pressure to the chin pushing down toward the floor. Observe the feelings as disclosed in his face and eyes.

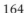

164

This exercise often relates to issues of submission, protest and surrender. Does the client engage playfully, fearfully, competitively, submissively, stubbornly? Discuss what you observe with your client and check your observations against your client's experience.

EXERCISE FIFTY-NINE: FOLLOWING

Either sitting or lying down, your client follows your finger with his eyes. You are weaving your finger back and forth at a comfortable focal distance for him, while pushing the limits of his visual frame. This exercise works to loosen the holding in the muscles of the eyes, releasing the eye block.

Chapter 24

The Oral Segment

Next to Irish setters, babies are the best at putting everything in their mouth. The baby's entire world is challenged by the question, "Is this something I might eat?" and frequently the world is found wanting. The mouth, a more sensitive, confronting investigative tool than eyes that watch without sensory contact, becomes the measure for the material world. It tests electrical cord, paper clips, paper dry and wet, stones, sticks, sand and grass by the handful. The mouth feels the metal and must decide whether to swallow or spit, while the eyes can dance over the object with delight and remain entertained but uncommitted. Even when the eyes express longing, it is the mouth that devours. The mouth gains support for its forceful undertakings from the chin, which expresses our wealth or poverty in aggression and determination. Our chin stands by or fails us in our self expression and needs.

Our eyes and mouth may disagree. Our eyes, for instance, may be cold and wary while our mouth is sensuous and open, or our eyes may be trusting while our mouth is grim. Before we learn to speak, we may depend on our eyes for interpersonal contact. With language, the oral segment becomes the focus for a powerful new self-expression. One of my students had gray, wary eyes, somewhat withdrawn, while his mouth was powerfully expressive and aggressive. He traced sensations in this area to early childhood. A single parent, his mother was working at a full-time job and had difficulty caring for him as well. When he was learning to speak at two years old, his mother moved back in with her parents where he was given constant attention and care. His eyes may have reflected his disappointment and consequent withdrawal in the face of his mother's absence during the first two years of his life. His mouth reflected the attention and encouragement he received with his grandparents and perhaps from his mother who was no longer struggling to work and care for him single-handed.

The oral segment joins the ocular at the occipital ridge. The oral segment's armor includes the musculature of the chin and mouth, the throat and the back of the skull, the occiput. Like our eyes, our mouth can reach out with longing or withdraw with anger. The mouth may be holding back angry biting, crying, sucking, grimacing and yelling. Our early history is suggested in our face which entices, masks, splits and subdivides in self-protection to sustain an ongoing relationship with the world. When working to open the oral block, we observe the various discrepancies that we read in the face between the eyes and mouth. We work for a congruent, open, fuller emotional expression. Are we able to trust our defenses to reestablish themselves when we need protection?

A client told me that after a full day of work, he invited his girlfriend over to his house. In the car driving home, he avidly anticipates the encounter, but when his girlfriend actually arrives, he feels encased and inaccessible. "Too much work," he mutters. In his case, because he does not have conscious access to his emotional history, we explore the contradictory feelings toward women. His eyes do not reveal his fear or his anger. Nor do they sparkle when his mouth smiles. His eyes are unchanging and indifferent; his jaw is clamped shut. Occasionally a humorous remark escapes like a bird from the jaws of a cat and his face erupts in a fleeting smile. In his situation, we theorized terrible early disappointments in intimacy that must be denied at all costs. Yet his hunger for intimacy has never died. He longs for contact but must refuse its promise.

EXERCISE SIXTY: PUSHING FOREHEAD AND JAW

Stand opposite your client and place your hand on his forehead. Tell him to look at you while he pushes his forehead against your hand and you push back. Then move your hand to his jaw and tell him to push against it. Both of you notice the difference in force and feelings and discuss the experiences.

To push on one client's forehead evokes a battle of wills which he clearly enjoys. With another client the forehead push evokes fear and collapse while the jaw push brings forth intense power in her eyes. Pushing her jaw becomes a battle of wills.

To what extent does this exercise contrast the ocular to the oral segment? The exercise often evokes a strong emotional response that can be understood only in ways unique to a particular client.

EXERCISE SIXTY-ONE: BREAKING THE MASK

In front of a mirror the client makes faces: bizarre faces, angry faces, absurdly happy faces, strange faces. She may accompany these faces with unintelligible sounds, loud and soft. Pay attention to the energy each face and sound evokes. Afterwards, discuss her experience and your observations.

EXERCISE SIXTY-TWO: LONGING

Instruct your client to lie down and breathe peacefully, while you sit in view nearby. After a bit, tell him to reach out with his arms as a small child might for his parent. Then have him reach out with his mouth by extending his lips. Encourage your client to make sucking noises.

Obviously this exercise evokes intense primitive feeling or powerful defenses against such feelings. It may be enough for some clients to discuss the defense against the expression of longing as an appropriate beginning.

As therapists, we need to be in touch with our own unmet needs. Some clients may frighten us with their needs. They may sense our fear unconsciously and push us sadistically with their neediness, or they may heroically protect us as they did their parents. Even as we imagine the possibility of doing this exercise with a client, we may catch a glimpse of dependence-autonomy and counter-transference issues lurking just beneath the surface. This exercise does touch into a basic primitive dimension of the therapist-client relationship which might better be addressed in another way.

EXERCISE SIXTY-THREE: MASSAGE FACE

Sit behind your client who is lying down and massage your client's face. Focus on the upper lip, the masseter muscles of the jaw, and the occipital ridge. Gently rock your client's head from side to side to encourage release in the neck. Cup the chin in your hand and open and close the mouth. Encourage the client to let you, the therapist, control the movement. Usually moving the chin reveals to clients how difficult it is for them to let go even when consciously choosing to. This exercise requires a sense of trust between you and your client. Consider carefully the transference and countertransference issues.

EXERCISE SIXTY-FOUR: GAGGING

As children we may have swallowed our parents ideas about life, what we should and shouldn't do. We ate all the peas on our plate whether we were hungry or not. Being force-fed ideas or food without adequate recourse to protest leaves visceral scars, tense inner tissue that cannot be reached through outer physical pressure. The throat and rectum are two ends of a primitive digestive tube and chronic contraction at mouth or anus interrupts the orgasm reflex. Constriction in our larynx can be alleviated through gagging, in which we vomit up the food and words we put down without protest for so many years.

As a technique, I recommend it only in the context of an ongoing therapy. The gag exercises are not recommended for people with a history of eating disorders.

Prepare your client for this exercise in advance. Tell him to come in with a relatively empty stomach. At the time of the exercise, your client drinks one or two glasses of warm water to protect his stomach during the process. Then near a basin or toilet the client gags himself with his finger, extending the finger slowly to the back of the throat to trigger the gag reflex. Tell him to be aware of feelings that arise and physical responses that follow the gagging process.

Chapter 25

The Cervical Segment

Then I started to find out about something that I'd completely
overlooked before, that every muscle in the head, the face,
the neck is fastened directly or indirectly to one or another
of the cervical vertebrae. It is quite impossible to organize
cervical vertebrae until you organized the muscles of the head
around the face and the inside of the face, and the inside of
the mouth, absolutely impossible.

Ida Rolf, *Ida Rolf Talks*

The neck or cervical segment, Reich's third segment, includes the
deep musculature of the neck and upper back, and the tongue,
which attaches onto the cervical bones. Reich's divisions have some
anatomical justifications, but were more determined by energetic
considerations that operate separately from anatomical structure.
The segments derive from what Reich experiences as a functional
unity of response in contraction or expansion. The platysma and
sternocleidomastoid muscles, in contraction, can block energetic
flow between the body and head. Tight necks can block crying out
in rage or pain. Long swan-like necks, thick bull necks, scrawny,
twisted, flabby, short and wistful, our necks conceal a resistance to
feeling that few suspect.

Reich witnessed a major breakthrough from working on a client's
neck in 1933. The patient resisted the disclosure of homosexual
fantasies, and that manifested in stiffness of his neck. By Reich's
application of pressure to the musculature of the neck, the man

suffered a severe physical and emotional response, a vegetative shock lasting for three days. He suffered from diarrhea, rapid heartbeat, changes of skin color, fatigue and pain in the neck and occiput. Such a reaction resulted from the release of what had been a continuous inhibition and damming up of biological energy, explained Reich.

From such an example it should be clear that working on the neck can have powerful results. Pressure through massage should be applied only on the sides or the back of the neck, not the front, to avoid cutting off the blood supply or injuring the larynx (voice box) and pharynx (air tube). Working on the deep musculature of the neck with clients seated or in a partial bendover position makes a crucial difference in reducing held tension. Because the musculature becomes "frozen" we lose feedback. As a corrective I press hard into the neck, to seek out the painful holding and apply a steady, tolerable pressure. The steady pressure allows the client the opportunity to relax the chronic holding now that feedback has been temporarily restored.

EXERCISE SIXTY-FIVE: THE GRIP

With your client in a partial bendover or seated, grasp the sides of his neck exploring for muscles contracted and in spasm. Apply gradual pressure to bring awareness. Tell your client to let you know if the pressure is too great. Too much pressure will cause your client to withdraw, a direct contradiction to the purpose of the exercise.

Also, your client can apply pressure to his own neck. With elbows facing out at right angles to the torso, your client makes fists and presses with his knuckles the sides of his neck. The client can also massage his neck, or relax it by placing a tightly rolled towel underneath his neck against the chair back while seated or the mat lying down.

Chapter 26

The Thoracic and
Diaphragmatic Segment

The chest and the diaphragm quite early in life begin to lose elasticity and movement as we resist shock by holding our breath and being deathly still. The intercostal muscles (those between adjacent ribs) grip our ribs in tiny vices, stiffening our chests in an expanded or contracted position. The thoracic segment includes the intercostals, the pectorals or large chest muscles, the deltoids or shoulder muscles and the muscles between the shoulder blades, armoring that expresses restraint and self-control at the price of core feeling.

Just below that, the fifth segment, the diaphragmatic segment, includes the diaphragm and the area beneath: the stomach, the solar plexus, pancreas, liver and the muscle bundles on either side of the thoracic vertebrae. The fifth segment contracts in a ring defined by the diaphragm over the epigastrium, along the lower ribs, and lower sternum connecting to the tenth, eleventh and twelfth thoracic vertebrae. When our diaphragm tightens, it is no longer the flexible sheath separating two body cavities, the upper and lower body. To open the chest means to increase the range of movement during the breath to a fuller, more natural expansion and contraction. By working to loosen the contracted musculature of the back and chest, we hope to restore flexibility. The concrete fixing of the chest holds back feeling, tears, rage, fear, longing and grief.

EXERCISE SIXTY-SIX: HANDS AND ELBOWS

The quickest route to opening the chest begins with loosening the back. Some people can only open up with softness; others ask for deep, insistent pressure. You must trust your instincts and check them out with your client. The goal is genuine contact. Sometimes a person's back is skinny with no fat. Every muscle seems stringy and unable to respond well to tactile pressure. Some clients have meaty thick muscles which defy invasion. Clients trained to endure may prove they are strong by resisting strong physical pressure. We must sense what will work or fail. As a therapist you may switch to soft work or interpret the resistance.

Your client lies face down over a cube of foam while you work on her back. Push in to feel the muscles on either side of the spine, the musculature at the base of the neck, the shoulders, and the musculature around the scapula. If your client feels nothing from your fingers pressed into her musculature, she may respond better to the gradual increase of pressure from your elbow. By establishing contact, you introduce feedback into a numb muscle structure. Be aware that one area may be numb, but an inch away the flesh may be very sensitive.

To make contact with a fragile, overly reactive body area, you must recognize how unpleasant and painful any touch may be. You may need to hover over an area so that your contact is purely energetic and the warmth of your hand elicits a positive response. Do not work in a way that splits the person from the body. Sustain a sensitive presence, expecting and demanding contact through intuitive touch or verbal response, so that your client does not become dissociated from the body area. Otherwise you are in danger of repeating a violation that may have caused the initial split.

EXERCISE SIXTY-SEVEN: OVER THE BARREL, STOOL OR BASKETBALL

Have the client go over the barrel, stool or basketball. The barrel provides stability and sufficient pressure against the rigid back. For more intense pressure, use the stool. The basketball is more specific in its area of pressure and less stable. Sitting on the floor, the client can get onto the barrel or basketball by pushing her back over the object as it rolls forward. When working with the stool your client must stand and lower herself backward over the stool. Be sure to stabilize the stool as your client mounts and dismounts it.

Assuming your client is using the barrel, allow her to explore the tightness of her back by controlling her position on the barrel. After she's made some initial acquaintance with the equipment, tell your client to stop the barrel at her upper back and neck in a position where her head and neck still rest on the barrel. Then ask her to roll the barrel slightly to feel the pull of muscles in her neck.

Ask your client to stop the barrel opposite her mid-back where the diaphragm attaches to the spine. Encourage your client to let down her pelvis as if to curl backward around the barrel. Ask her to report her experience. Ask your client to breathe deeply to expand and contract the rib cage. With each exhalation you can apply light pressure to the sternum or to the ribs on the sides, to encourage the corresponding contraction, but the pressure of lying over the equipment is often more than adequate. To bring energy to the whole body, your client goes up on the balls of her feet, pushing her pelvis up. This gesture will bring vibration to the legs.

While the barrel can be used to explore the extent of the lower back, the basketball fits exquisitely in the lower back when the client rests his shoulders, head and feet on the floor. This position relaxes the lower back and sacrum area, stimulating feeling in the lower abdomen.

Breathing Lying Down

Reich was not concerned primarily with armor but the full expression of feeling throughout the body. Having observed the breath being inhibited during inhalation and exhalation, Reich worked with the client's breathing to build energy that could be felt as it pressed against the contracted tissues. When the energetic emotional expression was unimpeded, the patient experienced the streaming of energy through the body. The patient experienced the build up of pleasurable sensations in the pelvis and his or her body was capable of release and surrender in the orgasm reflex.

This Reichian breathing process with the body-lying-down remains the most powerful method for gaining access to split off feeling. Forgotten memories surface; unique body states are experienced. To some Reichians, breathing, lying on the mat, is the only truly effective therapeutic bodywork for those who are capable of its rigor.

The therapist holds the patient very much like the mother holds the baby at a place before words where the expressive plasmatic movements and emotional attunement become the sole focus. Breathing lying down bypasses the egos defenses. Clients will regress, feeling dependent on and vulnerable toward the therapist. Some clients suffer from ambivalent feelings as the projected parent of their early life shares space with the therapist. If the client has a high functioning ego rigidly in place, lying down assists in accessing feeling that may be inaccessible sitting or standing up. If, however, the client suffers from early childhood injury exhibiting some schizoid, borderline or narcissistic features, lying down may not provide him with sufficient containment.

For some people, emotional release is tolerable only in the context of building ego structure. Clients with severe injury, without sufficient enlistment of ego strength, are more easily flooded with unscreened unconscious contents. Standing and grounding, working on boundaries, developing kinesthetic awareness and restructuring support containment and ego development as emotional release takes place. Lying down throws the client much more on the mercy of his or her unconscious life.

Some clients with very little ego resource feel at home on the biological ocean and easily row to safety in a tiny rowboat. With minimal ego defense, they feel comfortable in the grip of the unconscious. They are positive testimony for Reich's concept of the trustworthy core that underlies the persona and dark secondary layer of resistance. To other clients with insufficient ego structure, the unconscious is devouring and unpredictable, erupting in violent

176

storm, swallowing fishing vessels and their crews with ruthless indifference. To have this second group lie down and breathe for long periods is to jeopardize their functioning and sanity.

There is nothing romantic about a mental breakdown. Mostly it represents a journey that might better have been avoided because there is no guarantee that one can truly recover. Each client must be assessed in the light of the benefits and dangers of lying down, his or her relation to the unconscious and relative ego strength. Reich worked with some very disturbed clients. He was able to work with them five days a week for many months, providing them with profound therapeutic support. We may not be able to provide such support or possess Reich's remarkable gifts.

For those therapists that experience the trustworthy nature of the inner core, the Reichian breath process represents a powerful clearing process for dammed up sexual energy and repressed emotion (see exercise 18). But as therapists we must be cautioned not to make one technique answer every problem. For some clients, lying down will be the most natural way to melt the rigid chest and back, while to others, the posture will be unsafe, and enlist desperate defensive strategies. The therapist must listen to feedback from the client and have the wisdom to make cautious decisions concerning the use of such powerful techniques.

The model of silent observation sets the tone for all bodywork. The seated therapist and the reclining client are in different realities with a different time sensibility. The fifty minute hour may be too short a time frame to allow a client to breathe and process the experience afterward. The therapist may feel guilty collecting money while the client lies silently breathing with no guarantee that anything useful will emerge or be translatable into psychologise, the language that justifies our existence.

A good training program subjects us to the clients' experience so that we know how annoying a therapist can be who interrupts the powerful breathing experience. Any deepened contact with the unconscious calls for a different pace. The free association technique calls upon the same sensitivities for the therapist to observe. Sometimes the client is moved to places beyond words and speak-

177

ing violates the therapeutic experience. The therapist is called on to intuit and observe like a fisherman contentedly studying the water, sensing the fish in the eddy of the stream.

For some body therapists the breathing technique with the body-lying-down represents the frame in which all the work is done. If we use the technique, we must enter into that kind of awareness: we expect a whole world of experience to take place; this is not just another exercise among many.

We can work on the seven segments lying down, releasing the occipital holding, working the eyes, pressing the jaw, pressing on the neck, opening the chest, diaphragm, abdomen and pelvis. We can work for experience of streaming, for the motions of the body as it moves rhythmically alive and awake, experiencing pleasure and excitement. As therapists, we must understand our own counter transference issues and have our own sexual life in order, because the body-lying-down can be aroused and arousing. On the other hand, when talk is put aside, the breathing body becomes less directly engaged with the therapist, less personal and more self-involved. The release from the direct engagement with personality frees the therapist's attention to study in depth the powerful rhythms of the body as it reorganizes around the core self.

Chapter 27

Working with the Shoulders, Arms, and Hands to Access Feeling

I remember years ago, a boy of seven or eight in the waiting room of a clinic, where he was apparently brought against his will, systematically destroying an empty soda can, ripping it into strips of metal with his intense, tightly-muscled hands. I admired his self-contained expression of rage. It was the only form of protest available to him that would not bring him more trouble.

Our body-ego expresses itself through our developing shoulders, arms, and hands. With our arms we can defend ourselves, enforcing a boundary. We can push someone away, take things apart to explore them, use tools, or reach out for what we need. Many girls and some boys are discouraged from engaging their companions in active play. They do not wrestle, fight, punch, or push. How do we distinguish between unnecessary aggression and healthy, self-affirming sport? Some children are likely to lack confidence in their arms to protect themselves. Withheld anger and fear may chronically contract and deaden the muscular attachments of the scapula. Prevented from sliding loosely in a wide range of movement, the scapula stations itself resistively against the push and pull of social engagement.

If we are to engage with others intimately, our contact needs to extend easily from our hearts to our arms, our hands and eyes. If we have not been permitted to push people away, we are unlikely to feel safe enough to bring them close to us. We may long for them, dream of them, talk of them, but we are powerless to draw

179

them to us. Our arms are frozen. If people take it upon themselves to step in close, we are powerless to push them away or embrace them with feeling. We stand erect and distant or plead with eyes and smiles, but we cannot be in full energetic contact.

Our arms reaching up through the spine as an extension of our heart, head, and genitals are vital to deep intimacy. We would like to trust our strength to grasp situations that come upon us suddenly, to handle emotions, to put our finger on discrepancies, to shoulder our way in or elbow our way out. The following exercises help awaken energetic flows through shoulders, arms, and hands, essential pathways to maintaining good boundaries and accessing feeling.

EXERCISE SIXTY-EIGHT: PUSHING HANDS

You and your client face each other each with one foot forward. Your hands meet as you both push forward and pull back with your arms. This approach involves a rhythmic, playful engagement in which you are neither aggressively competitive nor withdrawn and rigid. Do not lock elbows, but allow a "give and take" interplay. The process tends to open the heart in relaxed contact. Explore your client's response to see if he meets you with fear, rigidity or force. The exercise allows for an understanding and correction of rigid responses.

EXERCISE SIXTY-NINE: LEANING AGAINST THE WALL

Direct your client to put her hands against the wall, lean into it and do a few pushups. In this way the client feels her arms connected to her torso and increases energy through her arms. The client moves her shoulders back and forth to feel the their connection with her arms. When cut off from the rest of the body, arms can feel weak and fragile. Tell your client to imagine energy welling up inside her, moving up her spine from her legs and from the overflow of her heart, and then her arms extending out from the trunk as its living expression. The arms then have the force of that larger self running through them. Also have the client do the exercise while thinking angry thoughts. Repeat the exercise with your client thinking loving thoughts. Notice energy shifts.

EXERCISE SEVENTY: VIBRATING ON ALL FOURS

Your client gets down on all fours on a comfortable rug. Tell him to feel the weight of his body pushing down and the solidity of his legs and knees as they support him. Direct your client to turn the fingers of both hands facing each other. Now the client does a few modest push-ups and pumps his arms gently with each inhale. The purpose is to establish a vibration in his arms and to sustain it for a while. Once the vibration starts, your client may stop the pumping movement unless the vibration ceases. With time, the vibration spreads into the shoulders, chest, and back. As with all exercises, discuss with the client any feelings or images that occur.

EXERCISE SEVENTY-ONE: SWING ARMS

Your client swings her arms vigorously for a few minutes forward and back, alternately, her hands swinging up to shoulder height. Instruct her to be aware of her shoulders moving, so that she feels them as separate from her neck and chest. This simple exercise powerfully reveals holding in the neck and shoulders. Also helpful for freeing the shoulders is the Cat Arch, exercise 40.

Chapter 28

Working with the Legs and Spine—
Repairing Our Brokenness

The spine is the central organizing structure of the body. We can feel our link with other vertebrates that, like ourselves, carry this chain of linked bones culminating in a head. For us human beings, the great triumph was standing up, accomplished by shortening the pelvis. By standing erect, we shifted our center of gravity from the diaphragm to the "hara," an inch or two below the belly button. The distance between those points represents our standing up, our mid-section, our third chakra of power, the solar plexus, that joining of the upper and the lower body in polarity and intense contradiction, lofty sky elements linked with the coarse, instinctual earth. Standing up we differentiated ourselves from nature and came into self expression.

Although we are addicted to locating ourselves in our head as if our intelligence kept no other dwelling, the spine represents a generous extension of intelligence manifesting like a god in different forms. We can kinesthetically experience the unifying presence of the spine while we ground the energy of our trunk through our legs. At the base of the spine is the sacrum, a bone formed from the fusion of five vertebrae, that transfers the body's weight to the hip joints and into the legs.

The spine is divided into five sections: the seven cervical (neck) vertebrae, the twelve thoracic (chest) vertebrae, five lumbar (pelvis) vertebrae,the sacrum, and the coccyx (the tail). I think of the spine like a whip, capable of incredible force when the energy is free to gather and travel the length unimpeded. If the flow is dammed up, the spine is weakened. We think of standing up as a time-specific developmental stage occurring at approximately the first birthday. However, the standing up stage not only involves the developmental awakening of key muscles in the legs and pelvis but also continues with the more gradual development of the lower, middle and upper back. To hold ourselves erect calls for a body evolution extending through childhood.

When we lose the power to protest, the continuity of the spine is broken or never develops. We no longer have backbone. With our self-expression curtailed, we weaken or we rigidly hold ourselves as if to deny our violation. If we are humiliated repeatedly early in life, our shaming organizes somatically in collapse at the diaphragm, making our spine bent and unstable as it reaches up to support the head. Where the cervical and thoracic vertebrae join, the body may build a thick platform as compensation to support the head. Huge bulky muscular columns may stand on either side of the lower spine in attempts to support what the spine fails to sustain.

Ambivalence in standing can be observed in the shifting signatures, the movement from the initial signature to shadow signature. Usually within the first five minutes of standing, a client will reveal her discomfort of standing as she makes the transition to a more established stance. the uncertainty of stance can also be seen in the shifting of spine from side to side. In standing up, we are often told not to "slump," to throw our shoulders back. The pectoral girdle, the scapula and clavicle, superimposed upon the ribs, visually confuse the issue.

The legs and spine must be continuous and kinesthetically awake in order for us to be embodied. The following exercises help to build one continuous energetic path from feet to head while standing up.

EXERCISE SEVENTY-TWO: BREATH AND VIBRATION

In this exercise we build an energetic track through the wilderness of feet, ankles and legs into the pelvis and abdomen, back and upper body. The first major goal is to establish uninhibited breathing and secondly to encourage a full body vibration, beginning in the legs, for approximately forty minutes. Your task as a therapist is to help clients survive the anxiety, minor pain, irritation, fear, intellectualizing or grandiosity that may threaten to take over the process of standing.

Have the client stand in the aligned position with bent knees. Encourage the client to breathe naturally and deeply. Some clients hold their breath in deathly stillness and others force their breathing. We are after "uninhibited" breathing. If the client experiences any severe response, stop the exercise. As a therapist, you must judge what "severe" means. The "seasoned" client, long acquainted with bioenergetic exercises, is ready to stand through the discomforts and fears that may arise until the second wind, when the pain eases and the client may feel pleasure and a sense that she could go on for ever. The client then experiences streaming which pervades the pelvis and gradually rises up through the body.

Start with a few ankle exercises and bring your client's attention to his legs, reporting to you how they feel. If the client is wearing shorts, you can see changes of coloring in the legs and observe in what areas the energy seems particularly cut off. Sometimes the knees are cold and can be rubbed or lightly touched to encourage energy flow. Tense thigh muscles can be gently pommeled to loosen the contractions. The feet and ankles can be massaged to frame in more arch and open the energetic field. You may direct your client in a bend-over to break up pain or tedium and help unify his upper and lower body.

After a few sessions, your client will experience a greater trust in his legs to support him, and his upper body will let go of its obsessive grasping after safety, a place to hold on. When your client is standing for long periods, it is useful for you to remember the eight stations to identify the energy blocks. If the energy is not moving in the legs, a neck exercise (station seven and eight) or a lower back exercise (station four) may make the difference.

Chapter 29

Energetic Release
in the Abdomen and Pelvis

Reich's sixth segment, the abdomen, includes the large abdominal muscles, the lateral muscles that run from the lower ribs to the upper edges of the pelvis, and the lower muscles of the back, the latissimus dorsi and sacro spinalis. The pelvis the seventh segment includes all the muscles of the pelvis and lower limbs. The midsection, a center of power is often constricted with fear developed from standing up in the world, from measuring ourselves against others. Here we find the activation of our desires being brought forth out of an unconscious world. The thick, supporting lumbar spine must bear the weight of what is taken on in the world.

The lumbar region suffers the frustration of middle management, caught between urges and adaptation. The feeling the upper body expresses in hitting or reaching out is different from the feeling expressed by the lower body in kicking or lovemaking. The loving of the genitals is different from the loving of the heart and the rage held in the back and chest issuing from the throat is different from the piercing and crushing gestures unleashed in the pelvis. The pelvis cannot execute soft pleasurable movements while withholding anger. Under duress the pelvis pushes and thrusts in a forced, unintegrated way lacking the lush movement of the whole organism building excitement.

The therapist needs the utmost sensitivity in working with the upper and lower abdomen, the sixth and seventh segments, which are vulnerable, intimate and well-defended. Without trust and sensitivity, the therapist can easily violate the client or be successfully blocked. Against rigid holding in the belly, gentleness is required. Unlike the tough frozen muscles of the shell of back, the soft underbelly holds off intrusion precariously. The upper abdomen appears more prepared to be touched without serious threat, but touching the lower belly brings up intimate feelings, sexual feelings and fears of sexual violation. For many people, any pelvic sensations feel sexual and ancient, forbidden feelings long outlawed from consciousness.

Prohibition against childhood masturbation is often named as the cause for the cessation of pelvic feeling, but more broadly, the open expression of a generalized sexual feeling of pleasure, so abundant in children, appears to threaten many adults. Pleasure carries with it a natural autonomy and freedom, but adults regiment the living bodies of children. They spank the moving pelvis. In response to this threat, the pelvic area is compressed: the contracted diaphragm presses from above, the contracted abdominal wall squeezes from in front, and the contraction of the pelvic floor pushes up from below. How is there to be room for the abdomen and pelvis to open to feeling? Breathing deeply lying down reaches into these levels of stillness and eventually awakens the deep, sacred feelings of flesh that lost or never achieved identification with self.

EXERCISE SEVENTY-THREE: OPENING AND CLOSING

Lying on the mat her knees up and feet placed closely together, your client opens and closes the knees in conjunction with her breath. With the inhalation your client opens her knees wide, allowing her legs to hang open to feel the stretch in the inner thigh muscles. The gracilis or "virginity muscles" often contract from unconscious fears of genital injury and block energy moving from the legs to the pelvis. With the exhalation your client brings the knees halfway towards vertical, and sustains the pressure on the inner muscles. The client continues the opening/closing movement until vibration is established. Direct her then to hold her legs in a place that maximizes the vibration. The exercise is often experienced as pleasurable.

EXERCISE SEVENTY-FOUR: PELVIS SEQUENCE

The sequence of these exercises is to be continuous so that when the client tires of one, she moves immediately to another. The exercises can be maintained in any order. Repeat them for thirty or forty minutes. Direct your client to begin by kicking on the mat, gently at first, then to kick passionately, intensely for a short period. The next exercise is to bounce the pelvis on the mat while her knees are up and feet flat. Thirdly, with feet flat on the mat, she lifts her pelvis up as high as possible raising her heels so that the balls of the feet and shoulders support her. Finally, tell her to lift her legs into the air, supporting her lower back and stomach muscles by putting a fist under her sacrum.

The Orgasm Reflex

Reich, in his efforts to open up sexual energy in his patients, stumbled upon the orgasm reflex, which became an important goal in Reichian therapy. Reich was the master of techniques that brought forth this body reflex, which presumably was the precursor to genital potency. Later therapists have been less successful in evoking the orgasm reflex, and genital potency has proven more independent of the reflex than expected.

For Reich anxiety centers in the upper body in the respiratory and cardiac region, while the vegetative center, the source of bio-electrical energy pushing from center to periphery, is located in the solar plexus and pelvic area, the lower body. The cardiovascular system pumps the fluids from the center to the periphery and back. Inhibited breathing is the principle repressive control that operates in a neurosis; it is a tyranny of the upper body over the radiating, creative pulsations emanating from the lower centers. In a healthy structure the whole body expands, contracts and discharges in response to the pressures of fluids and electrical charge. The pelvis is free to respond to the full pulsations of breath just as the upper body surrenders to the urgent life of the pelvis in orgasm.

The model for pulsation and release of tension is found in the growth of the cell. In the egg cell, growth through the intake of fluid is limited, until met by an energetic charge. Mechanical tension is joined by electrical charge. In the expansive process the membrane contracts opposing the pressure from within. The surface tension and internal pressure intensify and result in vibration and undulation. Rather than burst, the cell finds release by dividing, through which the same volume content is held by a larger membrane.

In orgasm, sexual tension builds in the heart and abdomen before concentrating in the genitals. Excitation increases until release during which involuntary contractions throughout the body musculature are accompanied by electrical discharge. Mechanical tension is joined by electrical charge moving toward discharge and mechanical relaxation, the orgasm formula discussed earlier. Failure to release completely is experienced as anxiety. Sexual dysfunction can be understood as an interruption of some aspect of the orgasm formula.

Working with the breath is essential to establishing the orgasm reflex. Clients often when lying down assume a forced breathing. Instead they should be encouraged to breathe naturally. The therapist notices if the client has an inhibited inhalation or exhalation. With the exhalation, the therapist can press in on the abdominal wall between the sternum and the umbilicus. The client is encouraged to tighten and release the pelvic floor, the muscles between the anus and genitals. These endeavors are in preparation for a simpler breathing exercise that supports the natural movements of the pelvis. The pelvis, Reich says, in the orgasm reflex, is not pushed forward by the thighs and abdomen but swings naturally forward with the exhalation. In an exercise, however, the movement of the pelvis can be assisted by a light pushing from the legs with each out breath.

For the following exercise I am indebted to Ed Svasta, a Bioenergetic Analyst.[1]

EXERCISE SEVENTY-FIVE: THE ORGASM REFLEX

With your client lying on her back, her knees up and legs comfortably apart, tell her to push her feet lightly against the floor with each exhalation. Her pelvis will swing forward (upward), and will drop down with the inhalation. Moving the pelvis in rhythm with the breathing helps to unify bodily movement. Work with resistances and inhibitions to the movements through light touch in areas where energy stops.

The exercise represents a basic release exercise helping to establish the correct pelvic movement. It should not be pursued as if the orgasm reflex were tied to it with a string.

Section Five

Embodiment and the Psyche-Soma Correspondence

Chapter 30

Embodiment—Being at Home

> Of course, one has to link the body to the self, because the
> distinct body is the distinct appearance of the self in three
> dimensional space. . . .
>
> C. G. Jung, *Nietzsche's Zarathustra*

If you are at home in your body, you can be at home anywhere.
Being at home is embodiment. Our embodiment carries with it a
great range of experience. The body can seem so ephemeral one
moment and leaden the next. Is the body a great encumbrance or
our best friend? Are we pushing against the limitations of our
clumsy senses or are we overcome by their brilliance? Whether we
have split our body six basic ways, seven Reichian ways or eight
standing ways, we are seldom so numb as to miss the elation of
stars in a night sky in the country or the intensity of chocolate
covered cherries. There is always something to hold onto in life
that is precious, even under the grimmest circumstances, like a
clean shirt or hot coffee when you are cold. And these precious
moments are simple body experiences with personal meaning, not
rarefied aesthetic or intellectual moments of uncovering truth.

On a somatic level, to be embodied means to break through the
character armor and establish a clear, energetic flow, to connect
the split off pieces so we are whole and in contact with ourselves
and others, what Reich described as the genital character. This is
in contrast to the neurotic character whose damned up sexual

energy prevents streaming energy and full sexual functioning. The genital character is emotionally present and spontaneous, sexually alive and physically vital, governed by a natural self-regulation rather than an unconscious compliance to rules. To Reich, Jesus was a genital character whose vibrant health healed others, accounting for many of the miracles.

Through defensive strategies of the psyche, we can deny the reality of our bodies and live in a fantasy state that suits our idea of life. We want to be special, not like everybody else. We don't want to see our dark side, our egocentricity, our fear or our rage. Split off from shadow nature, we imagine ourselves good and decent because it is intolerable for us to be other than heroic. How can we accept limits that bridle our imagined selves or cooperate with disciplines that define us so abruptly? Nonetheless, the body imposes limits and we function best with discipline. Our bodies humble us; they define us in ways that link us with others. In the metaphorical separation of our nature, our body is portrayed with base appetites as the improbable companion to our psyche-spirit self, as the stubborn burro or the dirty pig. Nevertheless, the body is not always stupid and coarse waiting for spirit for a glimpse of light. The body-psyche-spirit menage-a-trois is more complex and mysterious because the body soars, the body educates, the body guides, the body structures the reality that spirit enters.

As babies our psyche and soma cohere through the attention of the primary caretaker. Responding to a biologically coded structure, we gradually embody, finding the use and balance of each function. When our coding is interrupted through trauma, a developmental arrest prevents adequate embodiment. Being is not at home. Embodiment calls for subtle refinements of bodily movement and coordination. Severe trauma prevents basic functioning and leaves a gap where experiential knowledge should be. Character fills in gaps and structures our disembodiment. The body in recovery addresses the failures of development as well as character structure.

As addicts of every stripe, we long to escape the body's limitation in time and place. All of us are powerless to change our body's

character without help. Structurally, we are fated to su
and injury in a predetermined way. We will sprain the s
many times and stress the lumbar vertebrae when we si
twisting motion that characterized us as a teenager. If we are to
change, we must address the underlying images and the restricted
energy that patterns our physical life. Members of Twelve-Step Programs know that stopping addictive patterns does not mean recovery. Sobriety is an attitude, a life view that must reach every
dimension of our being. Being sober in a body adapted to being
drunk can only be a first stage of sobriety. While our habitual patterns can change through verbal therapy and recovery programs,
our bodies often hold on to the character remnants until directly
challenged through an informed bodywork.

In the spiritual history of mankind, a debate has existed between
those who feel that higher spiritual development and God's favor
excludes the devotee from painful injury in this world and those
who feel that God's favor may in fact lead us into devastating crisis for the sake of spiritual growth. In Job, a good man is brought
down to the most humiliating circumstances. His neighbors, who
think that God protects those whom He favors, assume that Job
has done something to "deserve" his pain. Instead one might argue
that by utilizing an exquisite alchemy of this world God refines
us. Because of God's presence, we awaken to our separation which
becomes intolerable. The greatest of us may be the one struck down.
Job through his painful stripping down became tested in the fire
of being. He stood up to God and demonstrated a nature that was
irreducible, the enduring self.

The enduring self, the philosophers stone, is not ours by birth,
but develops through trials of fire, a self that is trained to a flexible tenacity and positive vision. The enduring self, our identification with the soul, is a blade that cannot be sheathed in the world.
In its marriage with spirit, the enduring self is at odds with safety
and at home only moment by moment in the living body. The
great spirits have often driven the body up to its limits and beyond
in a powerful embodiment. Those of us with addictions will favor
an approach which sees adversity as a doorway to spiritual awak-

ening. Recovering people have had to face the false self again and again.

So when I talk of embodiment, I do not suggest that the embodied self is free of pain or conflict. The embodied self works to be free of the past, to be fully present, to avoid nothing, to be honest and direct. The embodied self is at home on the planet, not from an imagined exemption from the dangers of life, but through a complex acceptance of his or her destiny. The unexpected inner guide whose voice calls us to greater development disregards immediate comfort. Our embodiment is the alchemical process that transforms us in this world. Embodiment means giving up illusion, grandiosity, and specialness for the sake of an honest, grounded reality, genuine contact, relatedness and pleasure in the basic experiences of life.

Chapter 31

Healing the Psyche-Soma Split

> For the real value of a personality is always symbolized by a
> jewel, a treasure or something of the sort, because everything
> is centered round that central value which would be the self.
>
> C. G. Jung, *Nietzsche's Zarathustra*

We are likely to perceive others as a unity while maintaining a psyche-soma split within ourselves. The split is the shadow side of our embodied self. We notice in others how their body expresses their psychological state. We notice clammy hands and fear in someone else's eyes. How clear to us is the fumbling of the gawky, ungrounded high school youth or the Miss Perfect look of the girl too frightened to be different. We do not perceive others by splitting their physical characteristics from their psychological nature. With others we resolve discrepancies with an inattentive flick of fantasy's hand. With similar ease we can extend ourselves into the tools we use, sensing the nail slam into wood and the wheels of the car we drive grasp the pavement as we corner fast on a tight curve. Our imaginative kinesthetic sense extends and contracts our body being without reference to bodily dimensions. And yet without help we cannot breach the psyche-soma split within ourselves.

Embodiment represents our capacity to bring diverse internal and external elements into an organization called the self. How long can we tolerate the anxiety inherent in complexity? Splitting, as a primitive defense, diminishes anxiety, and as a cornerstone of character, reduces the world to manageable bits where we contain our lives through a necessary self-deception. In single-cell organisms, splitting for reproduction (mitosis) occurs mechanically as a way to reduce surface tension, suggesting a physiological basis of splitting to reduce anxiety.

Wilhelm Reich's working basis for resolving the psyche-soma split was orgone therapy. He theorized babies were born intact and whole, and splitting resulted from the impact of the restrictive outer world on the instinctual core of the expressive child. Freud described a period of splitting and dissociation before the child is gathered up into a unified structure with direction. In his theory of sexual development in children, Freud traces libidinal movement from dissociated impulses to an organized genitality. In 1909 at Clark University, Freud spoke of the "dissociated sexual life of children in which each separate instinct pursues its own acquisition of pleasure independently of all the rest" until "the separate instincts become subordinated to the dominance of the genital zone."[1]

In 1932 Sandor Ferenczi wrote in his clinical diary about a schizoid patient and her process of splitting. His client regressed to a childhood personality losing touch with the adult aspect of her self. While in his office, the patient worked through intense feelings suggestive of terrible early experiences; still the patient failed to improve. Fragmented without the internal adult aspect present, the patient's outbursts were futile and yet, reflected Ferenczi, "the cessation of the total-suffering and its replacement by fragments of suffering may bring ... relief ..."[2] Ferenczi's early investigations are supported by later clinical findings that emotional catharsis will not heal until the splitting is resolved.

The concept of splitting is fundamental to a psychology of the self. In dissociation, a more developed form of splitting, we simply lose touch with some aspect of self; at a later stage the ego develops repression as a way to manage disturbing elements of our nature. In Melanie Klein's view, splitting occurs with all infants early in development. For Klein, from the beginning the infant must ride the wild horses of instincts bareback, Freud's Eros and Thanatos, utilizing the primitive defenses of splitting, projection, introjection and projective identification to contain anxiety. The child splits off the dark feelings and projects them and introjects the good perceived in the external world.

Donald Winnicott, on the other hand, perceived the child and mother as an inseparable unit. The child initially cannot bring together person and body as a unit. Only the mother holds the child together as a connected self. The child is a belly connecting to a chest and head, to arms and legs and pelvis, all pieces unless the mother holds the child as one. If the mother does not know to support the head as she picks up the child, the head and trunk are not joined. The good-enough mother manages to hold the child comfortably as a unit until the child can do so itself.

In the first few months of life, the good-enough mother provides her child with the illusion of omnipotence. She sufficiently anticipates her baby's needs so that what the baby desires materializes in response to its demands. And where the fabric of understanding breaks down, the baby's emerging intelligence organizes to support the illusion. The child waiting to be fed can hear the mother's preparations in the kitchen and tolerate the waiting. For a few moments the baby mothers itself. The developing ego in time makes the transition from total dependence to partial dependence, establishing a personalized being and body, forming the rudiments of a self.

If the mother attends to the baby's body but cannot relate to the person, or relates to the person but feels awkward with the body aspect, then the psyche-soma does not join. The body is depersonalized, the psyche dissociated and ungrounded and the rudiments of self unformed. From the perspective of Object Relations, the afflicted self of early childhood is unable to gather itself. The self is fragmented, fragile, tentative, undeveloped, split. Primitive defenses, however, desperately attempt to sustain an some aspect of the self intact at any cost.

Ideally, a child who is well cared for early in life develops a clear sense between inner and outer reality and achieves a manageable compromise between the two worlds. On the one hand the child takes in the outer world for its own purposes and on the other hand must accommodate the self to the expectation of others. The early omnipotence gives way to the capacity to negotiate creatively across the boundary of skin between inside and outside. The child reveals the self through creative acts. The child with an awakening self-consciousness owns and fills out its body and personalizes its inner and outer images giving them meaning. A functional and durable self is a hard-won achievement, dependent on many factors outside our control.

It seems to me quite revolutionary to adopt Winnicott's low-key description of the baby in pieces, the idea that psyche and soma come together for the infant only because the mother holds it as a unit, until the organizing intelligence of the child is gradually able to gather to itself the rudiments of self. This concept brings into question the romantic assumption that psyche-soma, pictured as being innately whole and integrated, has been unnaturally split by a pathologically aggressive, exploitive western culture.

Heinz Kohut in many particulars agrees with Object Relations theory. While the newborn baby has a self, it is only through good parenting that a functional, durable self develops; "it is only within the matrix of the selfobjects that this self takes shape."[3] In Psychoanalysis, the search into the past represents the attempt to cut out past injury so that healthy tissue will no longer be "plagued by the pus of the pathogenic repressed. Psychoanalysis was only interested in the past in order to understand better the present."[4]

For Kohut the injured self lacks a sense of developmental continuity in time. As an older adult, says Kohut, we may be disturbed when we sense that we have not fulfilled our basic or "nuclear" program which holds our early ideals which press for fulfillment in tension against our range of skills. "Once the program is in place, then something clicks and we have a degree of autonomy; this degree of autonomy we call the self. It becomes a center of independent initiative that points to a future and has a destiny. It also has its own natural, unfeared decline and end."[5] For Kohut and Self Psychology, analysis of the past attempts to read the program called the nuclear self in order to provide a feeling of wholeness and historical continuity.

In both ego and self psychology, embodiment reorganizes toward a functional ego and a durable self. Functional mastery means disarming our failed strategies for new ego strategies that are appropriate to each particular life engagement, a capacity to assess each situation accurately for what it is. A functional body-ego means we have dismantled our dysfunctional defenses. Self-making, the integration of splits, and the reorganization of our way of being, are fundamental to a functional body-ego.

A durable sense of self extends beyond the demands of healthy childhood functioning. Many of us would be more than grateful for the integrated self of a supportive childhood; but a durable sense of self extends to the philosophers stone, that goal of alchemy which is imperishable, that which lasts, an observing, neutral self that does not seem man-made. A durable self exists past the passions and dramas of the moment, sometimes revealing itself through dream and vision.

The goals of a more modest psychology aims at developing a sense of self that can be trusted no matter how difficult the present moment. The enduring self knows that it can outlast every darkness, every suffering, no longer rigidly avoiding pain or fear of pain. A self that endures knows that the self is related to others, to life itself and to nature. Even in death, we are letting go to a nature that goes on. The sense of ourselves as a part of nature puts to rest the ego's struggle to be exempt and special. The surrender to life's processes is the mastery of the durable self whose nature like water, is modest, adaptable, relentless, and escapes the restrictive destiny of a single identity. The durable self affirms an object constancy, a sense of trust from one moment to the next, a pleasure in the unexpected nature of life. And the durable self may go on to experience mystical states, states of identification with nature and with the imperishable forms of God.

Chapter 32

Ambivalence and Embodiment

The energy that connects us to ourselves as an embodying, integrating force can become mired in ambivalence. We are born into a world of difference, of left and right, up and down, psyche and soma and light and dark. We become partial creators of the "good" and "bad" breast, and we gather all these differences to ourselves and coordinate them into a functional structure. Caught as we are in the center of so many polarities, we may be unable to proceed, to go left or right, marry or stay single, live in Colorado, New Hampshire or France, attend graduate school in economics or teach high school English. We may not know what pants to wear, what movie to see, what friends to develop. And when our lover, at our enticement, draws us close, we may be thrown into a terror that can only be quieted through distance.

Often our ambivalence can be traced to childhood injury specific to our present situation. A man reluctant to marry does not want to duplicate the terrible marriage of his parents or is hopelessly entangled in unresolved Oedipal issues. How understandable. How open to intervention. More difficult to work through is the ambivalence of the dysfunctional self that never found an early integration, whose care as an infant was inadequate so that psyche and soma never were felt as a unit and the good and bad object could never be held together. If we are to personalize our lives and have an embodied self, we must confront ambivalence, not necessarily to resolve it, but to embody it, to hold our dilemma in our two hands.

205

Ambivalence may serve us as an unconscious, childlike dependence, a passivity, an avoidance that forces others to take charge. There is no middle ground for certain choices. The middle is an avoidance. The middle is our ego-centricity.

"Do you like my dress?" she asks.

"Yes, its fine," he responds.

"If you don't like the dress, just tell me!" she says in exasperation.

"What's she so upset about!" he exclaims. He holds a middle ground that means "I don't care. Don't bother me." Sometimes we seduce our friends into taking sides to quell our anxiety and solve our problem. Ambivalence provokes rage in others towards us. They act out our unconscious rage while we remain cool and morally superior. The anger of others allows us to remain intact without having to feel split apart.

Possibly we are unwilling to accept limitation and face loss. All choices involve loss. For many people with terrible early and unremembered losses, one more loss is intolerable. If I choose to marry, I give up my small freedoms. If I choose marketing, I will never be the painter I dreamed I might be. It is as if the "perfect" choice will prevent loss, and every choice seems to have annoying flaws. It might happen that obsessive/compulsive traits are traced to a core ambivalence. I make lists and find myself unable to differentiate trivial considerations from significant ones. I cannot prioritize. Everything holds the same value for me. My defense against contact is ambivalence. My investment is in control. As long as we are ambivalent, the fantasy of unaccountability is maintained. There is, in fact, no way not to make a choice. We make choices, and experience losses even when we ostensibly make "no choice."

There are secondary gains when our ambivalent character develops a social network of concerned advisors who are played off against each other, a process which brings us a great deal of concerned attention. Perhaps we are caught between an old path and a new path, having not gathered sufficient energy and resource to place our feet in a new direction. Unconscious factors, such as the abandonment by our father, need time to resolve before we leave our abusive husband. Everyone wonders why we have not moved out yesterday.

Making important choices throws some clients into conflict. Ordinarily they find within themselves sufficient self to bite through. Mostly they agonize and decide until, one day, they are impaled by an ambivalence they cannot resolve. Perhaps they are not chronically ambivalent, but situational factors compound leaving them powerless to commit. In some cases the ambivalence is only the initial stage of an unraveling of self, a breakdown featuring anxiety, depression, a loss of meaning and somatic symptoms. With the breakdown of functioning, the ambivalence becomes one symptom among many.

In some cases, as therapists we must sit unhurried with our clients' stuckness and hold both sides of an ambivalence without buying into a hasty resolution. Chronically ambivalent clients may be enraged and disappointed with us. They have humiliated other helpers who ardently offered answers, but we have refused to help in that way. Of course, they must defeat anyone with quick answers, since they have been troubled for years with the problem. Someone else solving their problem will shame them. They make other people feel as powerless and frustrated as they felt in childhood while they play the role of superior parent. The therapist interprets these behaviors if possible in ways that do not humiliate the client.

How the body's ambivalence hooks up with psychological ambivalence may not always be clear. If the overlap is important for us to grasp consciously, then images will arise in dreams or during the bodywork. Counter-transference issues may be especially useful in this area. The failure to hookup the psyche and soma may not be the fault of the therapeutic understanding but central to the client's problem (viewed from Winnicott's model).

Theoretically we may explain chronic ambivalence as originating from a person's failure to form a cohesive self or to master instinctual impulses. Perhaps the ambivalence is a response to a developmental arrest that makes it difficult to proceed from an oral to an anal and onto a phallic stage or it represents an unresolved Oedipal conflict. Alternately, we may track our way back to an early splitting of the object. Ambivalence may also appear as a dissociation between the psyche and the body, an ongoing depersonalization.

Ambivalence can be dramatized by standing on one foot and then the other, by taking a step hesitantly forward and then back. We can encourage our ambivalent clients to stand in such a way as to portray their dalliance in life, their unpredictability. Their ambivalence can be observed in our gestures or purposely enacted. Knowing our clients' psychological ambivalence, we can see how their bodies allow for and are disturbed by indecisiveness. Unfortunately, the body's ambivalence, unallied with psychological disturbance, tends to go unnoticed. In the standing meditation, postural ambivalence can be studied.

EXERCISE SEVENTY-SIX: POSTURAL AMBIVALENCE

Your client stands for fifteen minutes. As therapist watch her move from initial signature to shadow signature. Mainly you watch her postural ambivalence, how the body may be unresolved about its twist to the right or left. You see the spine in trouble, supporting an upright position while toying with collapse. Notice the shoulders. Are they too rigidly held ever to experience ambivalence? Notice the little movements, the involuntary gestures and have the client consciously repeat them. Instruct your client to watch for inner movies. The task is not to do away with the ambivalence, but physically to feel the ambivalence through repeating small movements slowly.

EXERCISE SEVENTY-SEVEN: WALKING THE Y TIME LINE

"Two roads diverged in a yellow wood" wrote Robert Frost and the path he took was less travelled. We come to these forks in the road and our choice is most important. Your client stands at "the fork in the road" and describes the left hand path and then the right hand path. Bewildered by which way to go, your client describes what each choice might bring. Tell your client to take a step—which represents a year having passed—down the left hand path. Ask your client how he or she feels and what life is like. What losses are represented by this path and what gains? More steps are taken, with the steps representing larger increments of time. The client must then retrace his steps to the fork in the road and follow the same procedure down the right hand path. Retracing his steps, he may choose to step back into the past as well. By returning to the past down the stem of the Y, the roots of the dilemma can be explored. With each excursion the client must return to the present at the fork in the road. If no resolution can be obtained at this time, have the client return to the fork. Here he chooses to stay at this time. How does it feel to be here? What is he losing by staying here? What is he gaining? What injury cannot be healed yet? What aspect of self is preserved by staying stuck?

Chapter 33

Body

> But the body is, of course, also a concretization, or a function, of that unknown thing which produces the psyche as well as the body; the difference we make between the psyche and the body is artificial. It is done for the sake of a better understanding. In reality, there is nothing but a living body. That is the fact; and psyche is as much a living body as body is living psyche: it is just the same.
>
> C. G. Jung, *Nietzsche's Zarathustra*

To the question "what is body?" the mind spins. There are so many bodies. The body is a cultural construct, a manifestation of family, of imposed ideals, of shadow, of blocked and charged responses, of collective implications, of genetic peculiarities, of biological functions. Before intellectual investigation, the body evaporates to images. The body has been invisible for years unaddressed and ignored, left in the waiting room of the therapist's office. The body is ruled out of therapy because of the fears of sexual invasion, but also the body is absent because culturally the body is divorced from our spiritual salvation, divorced from our psychological and interpersonal development. The body is a cultural toy, a lure to entice a mate, an object to possess.

In the face of pervasive denial of the body, Reich anchored the psyche into the biological functioning of our body-being. His movement from a measurable libido to orgone, to the ether that sustains solar systems and life, opened up the biological body metaphor to the language of physics and religious thought. The human body as pulsing, sexed and vulnerable became a part of nature's cosmic and earthen cloth. Theorists since Reich have backed away from orgone, preferring the biological roots alone, removed from metaphysics. We are so conditioned not to see the bodily presence that we have to reduce our belief to the body as biology, as if science which measures us has the only real grasp of our bodily nature. We have forgotten that any measure is a metaphor; it is not the thing itself.

We have many physical bodies. Throughout our life the body keeps changing with twists, bends, straightenings, tightenings, and loosenings. We have a baby body, a child body, a teen-age body, a young adult body, a middle-aged and old body, a very old body and we tie these bodies together in photo albums. We laugh as we recognize ourselves and family members with and without hair and glasses. "You were such a cute kid," we say. From our childhood to our old age our various bodies may be dramatically different and yet, hold something recognizable of us as continuous being, a thread of nature stringing the beads of body. With all our body's differences, it is inspiring to see our nature emerging from each change of form.

How remarkable as well to see our son or daughter look exactly as we did at a particular age, a powerful genetic similarity extending through generations overriding boundaries of time, a genetic body regenerating itself with a life of its own. We see our family body not only as the genetic body but also the shared attitudes and mannerisms, the family's vocabulary of movement possibilities indelibly recorded. We have a characterological body, a defensive structure somatically and psychically held, and a core or energetic body, the liberated body that has stepped from the cave into the sun, alive, vibrant, vulnerable, passionate, responsive, receptive. We have also our animal body, instinctual, sexual.

And as if that were not sufficient, we have a body that extends beyond our physical boundary. Our hat, like our dog, looks like us. Our presence fills a room even in our absence, lingering at the opened briefcase and settling into our favorite chair. God forbid someone else should sit there in our presence. Our energetic body, a field that retains our limbs even after we lose them gives us pain in the foot blown off in war. And if reincarnation is true, we carry with us body patterns and predispositions we inevitably recreate with powerful unconscious intention in each new body home.

Who we are comes through shaping our changing form so that we are identifiable as a child and an old person. It can also be said that our bodies hold the unfoldment of a particular future; our bodies are coded for a particular destiny. The natural athlete finds it hard to avoid sports. With perfect pitch the development of music may be inevitable. And how do we deal with a biochemistry that favors obesity, alcoholism, depression or schizophrenia? Our bodies are not neutral, but lean on us, pushing us toward a doorway we may feel is not of our choosing. The body in its virulent form can kill us too soon or demand a painful discipline we would have given anything to avoid. Our body like death itself, becomes our teacher, a coded message from Creation in a language we have no choice but to hear.

In this book we have talked of the shadow body in relation to the ideal body and found techniques to explore the liberated body through postures that organize and plug into core energies. We may look to the transcendent body standing firmly on two feet in another realm leaning towards us occasionally to be felt and seen. It is ourselves in numinous form, essential to our enduring identity, with only the trick of consciousness holding us here, now. There is that divine twin, the shadow of the self, our intangible voice of being reflected in vision and dream—so many bodies, such natural abundance to provoke our fragile consciousness to integrate the mysterious components of our nature without judgements. When we talk of embodiment, we might ask what of the many bodies had we in mind? We may smile and gesture toward all of them with a generous sweep of our hand.

Chapter 34

Six Basic Body Divisions

> The baby is a belly joined on to a chest and has loose limbs
> and particularly a loose head: all these parts are gathered
> together by the mother who is holding the child, and in her
> hands they add up to one. In faulty handling the parts add
> up to more than one.
>
> D. W. Winnicott, *Psychotherapy and Human Relations*

To establish an intact body-self, we need to carry out two directives. We extend ourselves throughout all the parts of ourselves and we return to a center. As a gravitational center the hara, an inch below the belly button, has been long acclaimed. Certainly to walk from that center in our pelvis carries with it a grace and solidity. However the body's center represents more than a fixed point of dead weight. Walking from our heart we inspire, and from our back we resist. In a body where energy emanates, immobility is the precursor to death. Our body's energetic form has the capacity to gather itself, to shift and accommodate, to build, focus and release with miraculous force and abandon. At times the body appears to transmute into spirit. The great Indian warrior Crazy Horse, taunting the enemy with his courage, rode through a hail of bullets unharmed.

The brilliance of the body-self lies in its defiance of fixity and limitation. The great athletes pass through impenetrable walls like the four minute mile. The great spirits walk on water and heal the sick. We may prefer the right to the left side, or the head to the heart, but we have a responsibility to stay in a bodily continuity, to explore the body's genius and feel the full range of our somatic expression. Even as the healthy body centers itself with unthinking facility, we can shift our awareness to anchor at different location points.

Often we are compelled to disown some part of ourselves and make it shadow. Wherever the larger self locates, we need to be there to walk with its rhythms and sing its songs. We need to feel the density of its rushing tides and smell the sea and know the call of horns at night that mark its home. And yet to know the self in its wanderings through the shadow and light of the unconscious world does not serve to integrate us unless we are securely anchored in this physical reality. The body can be most helpful in integrating shadow.

Six basic divisions of the body form a framework for body healing and integration; they are left-right, front-back, inside-outside, head-rest of body, upper-lower, and trunk-extremities We are very likely to carry our shadow where we fail to see it, under clothes and also on our backs, behind us. If we have split off our needs or our anger, our backs will tell of these feelings. In the splitting of inside from outside, we are coaxed away from attending to our inner feelings, learning to attend to the demands of others; or we close ourselves off inside, withdrawn from the outer world. Our skin may respond quite differently from our internal organs, one or the other reactive to our anxiety or depression. Most obvious is the difference between our left and right sides. The right side deals with the world, carries our social aggression, while the left side holds our receptiveness, our softer feeling, a distinction readable in the left and right eyes. Sometimes that order is reversed. We need to look and engage the two sides to understand.

The head and torso split is often captured in the statement, "He is too much in his head." People cut off feeling by entering the rarefied world of intellect without extending down to contact the rest of the body that drags along like a unacknowledged guest. The barely tolerated body makes occasional demands which are begrudgingly fulfilled after delay. Often the body and the body's symptoms are drugged into silence. The split between the upper and lower body, the upper torso and pelvis, has been the classic way to manage our sexual feelings, though denial. We live with nice people in the upper body, a penthouse, and seldom descend to the low levels except when the lights are out. Others may act out their longing for contact by compulsive sexuality. A division less easily observed, the trunk can often be unrelated to the arms and legs that extend from it, and the joints of the body can sometimes gain our attention through the rigidity of someone's walk or the person's failure of basic coordination.

Even with our splitting, the body as a plurality extended in space with its differences, makes possible our consciousness. In his lectures on Nietzsche, C. G. Jung said,

> You see, inasmuch as the living body contains the secret of life, it is an intelligence. It is also a plurality which is gathered up in one mind, for the body is extended in space..., What you think with your head doesn't necessarily coincide with what you feel in your heart, and what your belly thinks is not what your mind thinks. The extension in space, therefore, creates a pluralistic quality in the mind. That is probably the reason why consciousness is possible.[1]

The six basic divisions provides a form to exercise consciousness and intelligence, to reconnect and rebalance ourselves. "We do not know the hour when the master returns," states a New Testament parable. Gazing wistfully into the sky demanding divine aid does not help. By owning all the parts of our being, we take charge of our lives. We feel our legs awaken and our arms reach out. To feel alive in our left and right side, our upper and lower body, to feel backed up rather than spineless brings pleasure into the core of our living.

Left-Right

> I should rather say that in my early years I had two left hands ... I do not know whether it is obvious to other people which is their own or others' right and left. In my case in my early years I had to think which was my right; no organic feeling

told me.... To the present day I still have to work out by their position, etc., which is other people's right or left hand ... it may be connected with the fact that in general I have a very poor feeling for space, which made the study of geometry and all kindred subjects impossible for me.[2]

Letter of Sigmund Freud to Wilhelm Fliess

The left-right division calls for an internal relatedness that orients us spatially in the outer world. The coordination of our left and right eyes give us depth perception. The left and right polarity represents innate internal differences and exercises our capacity to make choice and to accept limitation and loss. We are caught between the masculine and the feminine, between the active and the receptive, and between light and shadow.

We develop a functional preference for our left or right side early in life. With luck we learn to cross crawl, to move our left hand and right knee forward together, and follow that with our right hand and left knee, thereby integrating the left and right side. We learn to cross the mid-line in writing and drawing, coordinating the left and right hemispheres of the brain. Always in danger of interference through trauma, our motoric skills come due at key moments in development as we step into increasingly complex movements.

The left and right sides provide us with different internal experiences which may relate easily to each other or operate in contradiction. The left and right sides offer us options. With choice comes ambivalence and indecision. To choose forces us to accept limitation and loss. The left often holds the "feminine." It is the side considered receptive, emotionally vulnerable and available, intuitive, shy, open, related, interior, and artistic. The right holds the male energy, extroverted, dominant, aggressive, organizational, pragmatic, masked, independent, and the one who loves systems. The polarity sometimes reverses and we find the "male" energy on the left. What is remarkable about these "mystical" assumptions is how observable the difference is when we gaze alternately into the left and right eye.

The left holds the shadow physically, politically, and metaphorically. Left-handed people learn quickly the many ways in which the societal world constructs a right-handed reality. The left-hander drags the heel of his hand through the ink as he writes. The scissors don't cut because the blades torque open rather than press against each other. In Jung's alchemical account, the seeker after enlightenment stumbles into the left-handed way, represented by the fool, the dummling in fairy tales. It is the path which engages the rejected elements of our nature that, when integrated, break the drought and restore prosperity to the kingdom. The exhausted male-dominated hierarchy is infused with lightness, humor, artistry and feminine grace, wisdom and fecundity.

Freud, the brilliant, aging old king, has been accused of inhibiting the creativity of his followers. When psychoanalysis suffered from a drought, it took the left-handed path that called on the inferior, discarded, feminine elements for rebirth. The men did the "real" work of analysis working with adults, while some of the women analysts found their traditional place caring for children. And yet through Melanie Klein's work with children, Object Relations was born, and through Anna Freud, Ego Psychology found its home.

Through the left-hand path, we are liberated from old fixations and compulsions. We surrender to an arduous birth. The transformative images abound when we ground our whole being in our physical nature. We bring back into balance the polarities that sustain our multidimensional identity.

The following exercises assist us to explore the extent of our left-right nature.

EXERCISE SEVENTY-EIGHT: LEFT-RIGHT STANDING

Tell your client to stand, placing most of his weight on his left leg, and after a minute, to alternate to the right side. If one leg seems weaker, he explores postures that strengthen it. Then, ask your client to align the knee and foot by placing the knee directly over the foot. Ask your client to describe how the left and right side feels.

EXERCISE SEVENTY-NINE: DIFFERENT SIDES

Your client uses a mirror to look at her left and right eyes separately. Ask her to describe similarities and differences she sees. Similar to exercise 15, you walk slowly toward your client first on her left and then her right side. Describe what you see and feel. If one side is afraid, withdrawn, or inhibited in some way, stand at a distance from your client, just at the edge of safety, so that her feeling can be available without being overwhelming. Discuss feelings and images with her as they arise.

EXERCISE EIGHTY: SIDE AGAINST WALL

The client leans against a wall using his left and then right arm to support himself. Then have the client lean using the left and right shoulder. Ask your client to describe the differences. These exercises bring us closer to our body's function by observing differences. There is no guarantee that great insights will emerge, but the process is integrating on a body level. The exercises awaken kinesthetic awareness and clients build a sense of their connectedness.

EXERCISE EIGHTY-ONE: WEAK SIDE AWARENESS

Suggest your client spend a day using her less dominant side to carry out the functions traditionally ascribed to her dominant side. If one eye is strong and the other weak, your client might consider covering the strong eye for an hour or a day. What feelings emerge from the shift?

Front-Back

Although we stand in the center of a circle, we must face one direction and be blind to our backside. We go forward and leave our regrets and pleasures behind us. Time defines us as facing a future and turning our back to the past. We may envision our future without a cloud in the sky, but shrouded in darkness, our back may not exist for us. Perhaps we split the good from the bad to preserve what is precious. One side may twist back as if mired in the past, retreating. If the upper body tilts back reluctant to enter fully in the present, the head thrusts forward into the future to compensate.

We are not reminded of our backside by frequent glimpses in the mirror. Shutting our eyes, we can call up a picture of our front but not our back, while in picturing others, we are more likely to see the whole person. Our needs, our depression, our fear, our brokenness, our vulnerability, our failures of posture, our lack of backbone, all these factors and more are written openly on our backside. We manage to dress up our front to hide such weaknesses. If we could exist as a face and no back, perhaps we would prefer it for ourselves. With others we have no problem taking in the front and back, the persona and shadow of our friends. With others we are intrigued by the complexity of human nature, a graciousness we may not extend to ourselves.

And what is so terrible about our backs that they have lost our acceptance? Many people find aspects of the back the dramatic high point of their sexual lives. They like the curve of spine into buttocks and thighs. Perhaps we should not rule out parts of us that we fear have grown awkward and bulging. What has formed us as we are? Genetics? The It or the self? We might do better to join with our shadow and grow up. We might step past this sulking and angry desertion of body parts deemed shameful and unworthy. What part of us judges? Whose voice do we hear? Let that part write its meager opinions in our journal so that we do not disown the critic but integrate the voice. The critic should sit on the board of personal advisers but not as the chairman. With our failure to accept our past, we idealize the future which draws us from the present. We use the imagination to distort and co-opt the present. However, when our front and back come into balance with each other, the past and future dreams integrate so that we stay present.

EXERCISE EIGHTY-TWO: BACK-FRONT MIRROR

Using a hand mirror and a full length mirror, the client looks at his back and front. What does he notice? Note changes in his breathing, energy, grounding etc. as he examines himself.

EXERCISE EIGHTY-THREE: TURN YOUR BACK

If the client is worried about a personal issue, she is to imagine it embodied standing before her. Then she turns her back on it. How does she feel? What do you notice as the therapist? Tell her to turn back to face it. How does that feel to her?

Inside-Outside

If we trust and respect ourselves, we develop a relatedness between the inner and outer reality. When I have clients stand, I suggest that they close their eyes so that they will not be distracted by the outer world. They turn inward to attend to bodily feeling. Some of my clients hold the balance between the inner and outer world pretty well. Others dominate the outer world, watchful and aggressive, noticing details. Still others are inwardly dominated. They have not sufficiently engaged the outer world to challenge their imagined world with external reality.

Some of my clients are dominated by the outer world. They "fix" their faces to reflect the emotional states of others. Their eyes have walls. They do not feel their bodies, because their feelings have never been a major consideration in their compulsion to adapt to the expectations of others. They have the uncanny gift of seeing themselves from the outside. They are an object to themselves whose safety depends on compliance and attractiveness. They can be assertive. They can confront others. They can create elbow room for themselves and still never value their inner life. They can demand attention and demonstrate neediness with an edge of anger, desperate for intimacy "out there." Through achievement they can experience themselves as an identity but they are not on personal terms with themselves. They never learn to be at home, to be intimate with themselves.

When the early parenting is inadequate, a greater burden is placed on the baby's capacity to fabricate a self-sufficient internal world. A false self splits off from the body-self, perhaps not all at once but in a series of hairline fractures, in tiny ruptures of feeling. We develop synthetic feelings that shape to the environment, while our primitive, real feelings rot in prison. Lost are the intricate interchanges of childhood that refine our sensibility and judgement. Our humanity has no genetic protectors and must be patiently developed in the family. It is the personalizing psychic force of the inner life that gives meaning to the teeming outer world.

EXERCISE EIGHTY-FOUR: INNER-OUTER

The client closes his eyes. He opens them. He closes them and opens them again. Encourage him to take his time, to experience the transition from the inner to the outer and back again.

EXERCISE EIGHTY-FIVE: OPEN AND CLOSE

Standing, your client opens his arms wide as if to welcome the whole world. Then he closes down. He wraps his arms around himself. He turns away to the side. He may even crouch a little. Repeat the exercise. The therapist and the client discuss the experience.

Head-Trunk

When we "live" in our heads, we cut off from feeling. We live an abstract life with our shoulders and necks rigidly held. We live an abstract life where numbers and concepts replace the immediate world of the senses. We separate ourselves from direct impact. We delay experience and route it indirectly through the mind which feels safe in a tower of illusion. We tense our neck and shoulders. Tension in the occipital ridge and around the eyes and mouth affect what we see and say.

Recently, someone told a friend of mine that he appreciated her mind. "I'm so intrigued by that mind of yours." She was both flattered and disturbed by the remark, because her family brought her up to value intelligence above all else. She knew from bitter experience that an isolated intelligence was destructive to life. I knew that her splendid mind was accompanied by a wonderful heart. In embodiment we join the head, the heart and the genitals. Loving is not feeling or gushing or romance but an awareness that gives meaning, which may be as cool as a glass of water on a summer day. Like water, love fills the shape of what is needed. When the mind is not braced against the heart, we have vision in our words. Cut off from the heart, the world becomes a desert. The voice becomes as dry as an insect rubbing its legs.

One has to wonder what has driven us to abandon so much of our body. How is it that we can use our body like a car just to get around in? What alien force drove us to abandon the instinctual throbbing of our immediate hunger, so that invaded, we learned to live entirely underground without feeling the sun and the wind? Tilting the head to one side or lifting the chin an eighth of an inch is sufficient to cut out the world. Such violence to our nature appears to be most possible during the vulnerable childhood years.

Why does the head keep us up at night when the rest of our body wants to sleep? Who put the head in charge? The head becomes a compulsive machine refusing to negotiate for balance with other body members. In the past, some tyrants were beheaded. Their contempt for others was aptly rewarded. The head can never be truly present without the heart open to ground in the miraculous world of the ordinary.

The pelvis has more world in it than we can imagine. In its depths live the holy water of the unconscious where great gods dwell, where imagination takes form and life springs upon us like a panther. We had best attend to the pelvis and listen to its belly rumbles. Unlock the hinge in the lower back where the muscles contract and release feeling. Let the pelvis swing forward without pushing. Let the pelvis circle as if some faint Brazilian wind has awakened a slow, steamy music of early evening. Let go of the north which so often is ruled by tasteless food, where people bundle up like shapeless pillows and shiver, taking careful steps on the ice. Embodiment calls us out.

Head-body balance gives us the capacity to embrace all our experience. Our head integrates with feeling and instinctual life, affirming our right to exist.

EXERCISE EIGHTY-SIX: THE TILTED HEAD

Notice if your client tilts her head. If she does, tilt her head a little more in the same direction of the tilt. Then reverse the posture. Ask your client how each new position feels. Have her look in the mirror to observe the tilt and the changes in position you prescribe. Does what she see agree with her kinesthetic awareness of the positions?

Upper-Lower

To be cut off from one's pelvis is to lose ground, to fail to stand in oneself, and to dissociate oneself from a feared animal nature lurking in shadow. We suppress its hungers which explode unexpectedly or leak out unconsciously. We project our dark nature onto others. The prurient news and the pornographic industry feeds on our split, while the madonna and whore speak of our failure to integrate the good and bad mother and achieve object constancy. A major function of ego remains unresolved. We have cut off from our sexuality and also from the dark rage we felt in childhood. We provoke our own deep fears by placing our split off rage onto another person, an "enemy." We are prepared to be punished by life.

Usually the second half of a successful body analysis liberates the pelvis. The head and heart must first be open. We have worked on the chest. We have worked on grounding. We work to open the belly through breath and touch. Through grounding on the body-standing-up, we bring energy up through the floor, through the legs to the pelvis. With the body-lying-down we work on protest and surrender. We bounce the pelvis, hold it up, breath into it, witness its movements. We relate the pelvis to the upper body pulses, to breath and heart beat, and to the body movement as a whole. We locate ourselves in our pelvis, in its tenderness and bulk. The primitive food tube that runs through us circles upon itself as it lies down in the pelvis. It gathers to itself tensions that often release when other parts of the body are touched. According to Gerda Boyesen, the sounds from the viscera instruct us in our efforts.

In a sex-negative culture, sex literature flourishes. Sometimes we cannot feel sexual toward those we love or love those we have sex with. Our sexuality is a product of excitement and the mandate of biology, orgiastic and indiscriminant. Why should our sexuality be curtailed by heart considerations or an ethical mind? Nowhere does the embrace of shadow have more urgency than the integration of the upper and lower nature where the amoral split leaves us at the mercy of sex and aggression. Instinctual life should be carefully integrated through family, education and ritual initiation. The hope of nature being innately civilized does not play out well in a world that pulls us to the lowest level we can attain. Cut off from the pelvis, every illness is not only possible but inevitable.

Without the energetic pleasure and joy of our lower nature in relationship, we suffer a despair that takes a thousand forms. Healing the upper-lower body split we integrate our "higher" and "lower" natures, our mind\heart with our instinct.

EXERCISE EIGHT-SEVEN: MOVING THE PELVIS

Standing, your client moves his pelvis forward and back and then from side to side. Discuss with your client how he holds back. After this, tell him to reduce the pelvic action to the specific movement that exposes his holding. Discuss this second experience.

Trunk-Extremities

The loss of our arms and legs would reduce us to a state of extreme dependency like a baby in the first few months of life, and so the splitting off of arms and legs suggest frustrations and abandonments during the first few months of life, although, clearly, the arms and legs take years to fully develop.

Without our arms we may feel incapable of defending ourselves. Perhaps as we struggled to develop function in our arms, a well-meaning parent repeatedly brushed our arms aside to clean our face or change our diaper. We might have cut off feeling early on, because we felt rage and feared to use our arms to strike or our legs to kick. We may have tried early to stand up just to escape the extreme dependency that felt so unsafe to us. We may have cut off feeling, particularly the feeling of vulnerability and weakness in our legs. We could not afford to give in to pain and fear.

To feel the helplessness of the earliest stages, we can lie down on our backs and make vague gestures with arms and legs in empathic replication of a baby. Perhaps we cannot see very well. We become fascinated by our fingers. Where did they come from? When we locate our feeling of helplessness, perhaps then we can try to grasp someone's hand as it extends to us, or we turn ourselves over with our legs and feet only. When we have felt the powerlessness, we can tentatively explore movements that begin our functional lives toward autonomy.

It is normal to feel powerless. The infant wards off this catastrophic awareness through an omnipotent defense. Gradually, with enough needs met, a well cared for infant begins to tolerate the feeling of frustration and anger at being small and helpless. It is able to "borrow" a sense of self initially, only slowly awakening to the truth as it develops. If, on the other hand, the infant were not so protected from the cruel truth of its powerlessness, we may never have learned to surrender to its proper human limitations. Grounding exercises are effective in working through disconnections from our legs, and boundary exercises in which we push away or push against a person or a wall are useful for our arms. Connecting the trunk with our extremities moves us out of dependence into autonomy. We develop a functional and durable self that engages others and through movement, confirms us in space and time.

Chapter 35

The Embodied Voice

Lately I have been listening to people's "voice" in therapy—their way of relating themselves to themselves, their observations and complaints—and have been drawn to the conclusion that one great asset of therapy is to help someone develop a consistent, continuous voice in the world regardless of their life going well or badly; the voice as it develops is not merely a voice of persona but it speaks out of the embodied self.

Even when thin, small and terrified like a scratch on the wall, our voice continues to connect each moment with the next and relates us to all the elements of ourselves. Such a thread, which might lead us out of a labyrinth from the savage self to the integrated self, is the fragile victory of our developed humanity which insistently functions as a faith, a belief in an organizing intelligence. Our voice is a voice over time associated with civilization, order and reason, even as it takes note of disorder, despair and ruin. Voice is closer to smell than sight; it is anchored in breathing and vibration, is interior and felt, and is sufficiently complex and embodied to ground us in blood and muscle as well as thought.

The voice developed past a mechanistic persona becomes authentic and modest in its self account, touching us with our common humanity. Listening to such a voice in my client, I do not intercede. Painful predicaments appear enhanced and vibrant. A deep listening like a silence takes me over. What solution could bring more to my client at this time than the depth of this dilemma held with such consciousness? Like a rope of smoke, we can use voice to lift out of the deepest pits. David as a youth sang to Saul and released him from agonizing depression. And Orpheus charmed nature around him to total attention as he sang.

I for one am visual and sometimes see images and energy as I work. All the more powerful then to me to hear a person's voice and then his embodied voice. The outer voice is perhaps shallow, disconnected and thin, interrupted rather than sustained through breath, but the underlying voice has a larger metaphor behind it and represents a posture in the world, a core signature, which adjusts its stance to engage particular events. An analytic body-work dissolves the discrepancy between an inner and outer voice and brings forward a more fully embodied attention.

Chapter 36

Embodiment and Wilderness Man

> Once out of nature I shall never take
> My bodily form from any natural thing,
> But such a form as Grecian goldsmiths make
> Of hammered gold and gold enamelling
> To keep a drowsy Emperor awake;
> Or set upon a golden bough to sing
> To lords and ladies of Byzantium
> Of what is past, or passing, or to come.
> William Butler Yeats, "Sailing To Byzantium"

A few years ago, I had the opportunity to visit Jung's wilderness haunt on the lake at Bollingen, a turreted castle part of which he had built with his own hands. The building expanded as a symbol of Jung's internal development. Reading about its stone floors and narrow windows, I learned of rooms where someone from an earlier century would find nothing to jar his consciousness. I saw in this reversion to earlier times a psychic, primitive wilderness where ghostly intruders could be distinctly heard. Jung would retreat to this haven from his busy Kusnacht home and find refuge undisturbed. I was somewhat shocked to discover on my visit, that Bollingen, while a relatively sedate village, was hardly wilderness. From his house, I looked across the lake and saw cultivation. The surrounding land was manicured and public. In contrast, for years the wilderness for Americans was immeasurable, through which men like relentless ants made arbitrary, rude paths.

Through the centuries, people tainted by a perverted culture have fantasized about the natural man, the wilderness man, about children brought up by wolves or by "natives." Society, some thought, corrupted the innate innocence of human nature. The law created prostitutes. In contrast, others thought that culture tamed violent passions. When Dr. Jekyll finally got in touch with his animal side, Mr. Hyde, he was compelled like an addict to transform into a body more powerful than his former ethical self.

Even as Americans we have reason no longer to be romantics about the wilderness. We have looked into the jungle of the heart, read of mass murderers calmly interviewed, and seen the face of Manson in his imperturbable righteousness acting as a mirror to humankind's unacknowledged cruelty. Some of our pure young men were sent off with guns so light and easy to shoot that you could hardly stop them. Some of them returned to a divided country insulted, deeply wounded, unhonored, in retreat, guarded, addicted, unfixable as a plastic toy.

While the American soul has been fed on the vision of a unending wilderness to exploit limitless expanding markets of opportunity, we have, as an extroverted culture, been drawn inevitably to the recesses of wilderness in the mind and body, drawn to Bollingen, drawn to Native Americans. In our fantasy, wilderness men are sages, models of embodiment, who live in round houses instead of square, look with eyes which see from the heart, speak with lips that are not thin and cruel, and possess bodies attuned to the earth. John Muir, who could walk off into the wilderness with a long dark coat, a piece of bread and a knife, inured to the cold and aloneness, discovered that there were cathedrals in the stones and giant trees—that nature was indeed sacred. He needed no imported Greek gods to fill his heart with inner mystery.

It is as easy as turning around to find an American who knows of the mystic unity of the wilds and prefers it to church. Imprisoned by culture, Americans have exercised the option of a retreat into the woods to find soul. The chosen people were led into the wilderness as a purification before they could enter the promised land. For some Americans, a romanticized wilderness, like the romanticized body, is the promised land. The wilderness represents what is unspoiled, undeveloped, outside the deadly shadow of humanity, open to creative expression and work, a test for heroes, where a person's authority is innate and unchecked, and she knows a natural state of awe and expansive pleasure. For some the wilderness is considered benign, like the romanticized unconscious, in which therapy is "in fashion" and the anguish of mental illness is seen as a great adventure.

After all the centuries of brilliant minds, of saints and statesmen and the protests of citizens, our dangerous nature is uncontained. With ferocity, we attack what we claim to revere. Across the globe we hear of the destruction of the rain forest and of whole species decimated. Oxygen is lost, ozone layers corrupted and indigenous populations are shot down. Our voracious species MacDonaldizes universes, while many of us pray to God that Nature with its devas and animal forms will forgive us at Findhorn. As a culture we have colonized and exploited, and then idealized what we have destroyed.

If the unconscious is plundered as an idealized wilderness, so are our bodies which are plotted against, constricted and starved, cut down, our omnipotence broken by riding our body to the ground. We exploit our idealizations. We do not realize that the body wilderness is sacred rather than ideal. Naked or clothed, we paste it to a wall. We drive it like a car. We do not know how or why the body wilderness works as, with inexhaustible tolerance, our bodies bend to our youthful will. Later, we put our bodies to sleep with drugs so that their true voices cannot accuse us in pain. Reich knew that alienated from our body wilderness, from our genitals, we became destructive of others and cut off from the energy of the universe. Having replaced the sacred with the ideal, we hunger for our inner wilderness man, the kingdom within us, the promised land. Rousseau dreamed of the ideal man of nature who is self-regulating, killing only what he needs, patient, unwasteful, curious, an intelligent animal. Reich's genital man, represents a sacred nature. The ideal is illusive and unobtainable; the sacred is dishonored yet always present with us.

Brought up in Africa, Lauren Van der Post (in an article on the wilderness) writes how he had the good fortune to live with the First People for three-and-one-half years. His account of the African bushman represents the best aspects of primitive man in nature. In this idealization we do not hear of the diseases, the curses that kill, the petty slanders that occupy the lives of all people, but we are told something important that does ring true.

> They committed themselves to nature as a fish to the sea and nature was kinder to them by far than any civilization ever was. The one outstanding characteristic of these people as I knew them, and which distinguished them from us, was that wherever they went, they felt they were known. The staggering loss of identity and meaning that we in the modern world experience was unknown to them. . . .[1]

Having lost the true and sacred wilderness within ourselves, we are lonely and destructive. Robert Lawlor, in his account of the Australian aborigines, says that their identity is not tied to possessions or boundaries in the tradition of western man nor do they look to a transcendent god. As wanderers on the sacred earth, free of enclosed spaces, their identity is taken from the place of their birth, their true mother, where they learned the legends and rituals associated with that specific area.[2] The bushmen and the aborigines do not suffer from living an abstract disembodied life. They do not presume to be better than the earth nor do they consider it a prison.

We are born into a brilliant, extroverted culture breeding a lonely people. Ill-at-ease in our bodies, we hesitate to set foot into the wilderness that could heal us. For us the birds, the moon and stars have no names. We have no family. We lose poetry and cannot sustain a generous story about ourselves. We have no cosmology to connect earth and sky, no heart that binds us to the sun. How can we be initiated into the wilderness of our bodies and ride the river of sexuality and dream great dreams when we have held back from our relationship to all living things? And yet we can hope that having entered the wilderness of being though any door, we must inevitably learn the sacred truths and feel the miraculous within the mundane.

Chapter 37

Character and Uniqueness

At the very heart of therapy, says James Hillman, is the need to experience and be seen in one's uniqueness. The unreflected use of any typology which generalizes people and fits them into a conceptual frame blinds us to a person's particular nature. Hillman challenges the analysts who mechanically apply Jungian typology to their clients.

> For if there is one thing each patient needs, it is to be perceived in his or her uniqueness and if there is one thing an analyst struggles with unrelentingly, it is to espy a particular and different self in each patient, the desire to see and the need to be seen cannot be overestimated....[1]

Unfortunately we can reduce the purpose of our work to identifying character or being attentive to the biological flow of the body while the client walks away, unseen. We can classify and treat a borderline character disorder according to established guidelines in an apparently faultless professional manner and fail to see more than the type. Some of us have experienced the emotional death of having been unseen in childhood. Those injuries to the early self, faithfully recorded in tissue, can be addressed by the therapist with the same inattention to the individual as the parents who inadvertently administered the original wound.

To be unique is to stand in our aloneness, in our unknownness without the layers of assumed identity to make us familiar to ourselves and anchor us in the mundane images of the world. Character is just one of the layers we mistakenly call ourselves. After all, we may identify ourselves nationally as American, regionally as Eastern, as a class member, as an age group, as a member of a special group like Baptist or Marine. We identify as members of a family that has its own curious distinctiveness. We identify our position in the family as youngest son or father. As a body we also know who we are: athletic, beautiful, wrinkled, ugly, uncoordinated, inept or tense. We like to see ourselves as heroes and heroines and then confuse our mythic vision with who we are, just another convincing self-disguise.

We carry with us our father's laugh, our mother's politics, a manner of talking and the phrases of our teachers and friends. If we let each layer go, who would be there? Could we tolerate the silence? We would have to be able to tolerate being alone. "Maturity and the capacity to be alone," according to Winnicott, "implies that the individual has had the chance through good-enough mothering to build up a belief in a benign environment."[2]

If we are to strip away character, we must work with a psychology of the self that is reparative of early childhood damage so that we achieve a sense of well-being sufficient to support our separateness and our uniqueness. The divisions of the body self need gentle movements to build relatedness. Kinesthetic awareness becomes more important than catharsis.

We need movements that help us feel whole, that identify our left and right sides and help us sort out our inside response from outside expectation. The child must be able to be alone in the safety of the mother's presence, able to gather itself or let go without interference, to discover its personal nature. Long silences in therapy may not always be resistance but instead, moments of reparation during which the client in the safety of the therapist's presence is able to experience the personal nature of his or her self.

From a body perspective, how can we assume that after each layer is peeled and until the final identity falls away, that any self remains? Perhaps a mere biology is the core and streaming is the closest we come to soul. Or is there some presence sufficiently undeniable that invades all the space of us that remains, even in death? With our attempts at being special, can we ever trust a word like "unique" to be free of the ego's manipulations? If we identify our "uniqueness," we will imitate ourselves being unique. Our uniqueness is the very thing we cannot see in the mirror but that others see. Yet our uniqueness is lived by us as we let go of identities and experience our place in life as embodied.

Archetypal experience connects us to life without the separateness that makes us special. A client sees in my garden a black cat staring fixedly into a patch of daisies, transfixed by some movement invisible to both of us, and she laughs as her mood shifts. Later toward evening I see a tree like a webbed black hand held up quietly against the red sky. It seems like a tree I might see anywhere on earth at any time and I feel comforted by its beauty and its permanence through change. My life may change but I will be able to see this tree again. The tree connects me to an unknown center where I am on a perimeter with no sense of being diminished. No wonder Jung was fascinated with the archetypes, the universal patterns which make up the vocabulary of images which structure the world.

No matter how insistently we clutch our specialness to us, we only feel more isolated, divorced and separate. Like the monkey who sticks his hand in a jar of rice and by grabbing is unable to withdraw his bulky fist, so our character bunches up as we hold on to everything that makes us special. Our uniqueness is not available to us in that way. Recently, on Halloween, I saw some friends with their faces painted, and I didn't recognize them at first. The contour of their faces were emphasized and yet every personal reference point was erased. Our bodies make movements that are simple, universal, archetypal or they make cramped, artificial movements full of self doubt, contradiction and dissociation.

When we let go of our ego-driven self, we experience life directly. We experience our connectedness, and uniqueness is hardly our concern. Momentarily our movements are inevitable and universal, and spirit and flesh are one thread from which the whole world has been woven. Our being evades all our efforts because we would name it and take over its sacred nature and force it to dance like a trained bear. Our true being may want to be seen but only on its own terms. It has reason enough to be afraid of the ego's "civilized" intentions.

William Faulkner tells a story about a boy's meeting with an archetype of the self and how he must let go of every vestige of ego. In *The Bear,* men meet each year to hunt, and towering over all other challenges is the hunt for a huge bear whose paw is marked by the injury from a trap. The bear, so old and clever as to elude generations of dogs and men, speaks of an older time before the great forests were hacked mindlessly away by puny, unheroic men. A boy, after several years of hunting, seeks finally to meet the bear and is instructed by an Indian. If the boy wishes to see the bear, the Indian counsels, he must let go of everything, certainly his gun but also his compass and his knife. The boy sets out as told. Only then does the bear choose to come close enough to be seen by the boy. The air grows heavy, the forest suddenly silent, and the boy watches a great muddy paw print gradually fill with water.

Chapter 38

Developing a Vocabulary of Movement

It's hard to realize exactly how stifled our body movement is. When we went to school, we were trained to sit in hard chairs for what seemed like endless periods of time. We squirmed and twisted and our bodies adjusted to a sedate life. When we were encouraged in movement, we learned a few body disciplines: a way to hold and swing a tennis racket, a way to dribble and make a jump shot from mid-court. We developed a limited vocabulary of coordinated movements which reflects mainly a cultural intention to support health and social cooperation, a general movement rather than one that might bring home to us the delicate framework of our particular physical being. We learned to raise our hand to speak, to throw a ball, to ride a bike, to stand in line, and to park a car.

Complex and gripping as these movements are, they establish us only as a collective being and do nothing to help us develop a sense of our particularity. Nevertheless, on the positive side kinesthetically, we have developed a solid ground floor of coordination in a collective vocabulary which relates us rather than isolates. There are demanding trainings like dance, sports, and martial arts which guide us to a more individual style of gesture and balance. These movements develop in us a sense of ourselves as sturdy in a present world, but we may never awaken to a unique language. We may live on borrowed movements; we may be well trained and genetically the carrier of natural ability, but supremely inattentive to the inner voice of self. With the exception of the few, in the world of embodied kinesthetic knowing, we are an insensitive and undeveloped culture.

I have asked some clients to make movements which derived from a sense of pleasure. I asked them to proceed very gradually and slowly, because one major way we override any experience of feeling is to execute a movement rapidly. For many, an unstructured exercise about movements of pleasure was too threatening to carry out. Some filled out the exercise with stylized movements from martial arts or stretching exercises. Frequently, clients run through a set vocabulary of movement which has reassured them in the past.

Little routines of movement reassure us, like rehearsed speeches. We have no occasion to experience spontaneous core movement and so our core signature remains unknown to us. (I am aware that what I call "core movement" is similar or identical to what is called "authentic movement," a recent development in dance therapy.) How are we to know ourselves unless we walk past the meagre repetitions of the shadow signature and the family gestures? Spontaneous, individuated movement need not be relegated to dancers and talented athletes alone. The key to finding such movement in ourselves begins with awakening to the pleasure of the simplest body movements and learning to be at home with ourselves, BEING at home, embodied.

The routines we have learned can lead us to a developed body intelligence and to a kinesthetic knowing. At one time or another, many of us have discovered that our bodies remember what we consciously have forgotten. Our hands play a piano piece which we have no memory of. Our feet carry us to a place, but we hardly remember how. The body drives the car home with us barely present. Kinesthetically, we remember and know. Knowing is not reasoned. Our hands know where the tension and pain is when we touch our clients. We learn to listen to and leave room for this body intelligence, allowing our kinesthetic knowing to lead us.

Also in characterologically restricted places, we might develop a vocabulary of movement, a dance, a kata, to lead us out of somatic darkness, but never a harsh dance, never to abolish darkness, but to provide a somatic ladder into a freer dimension. For instance, we may crouch down and then stand and open our body, our arms outstretched. We walk on our heels nonchalantly and then on the balls of our feet aggressively. We test the limits of our nature working with our polarities. We carry on a kinesthetic dialogue between the left and right sides, the front and back, the upper and lower halves, and our shadow and ideal body, until we come to a new understanding that the body has found.

Our physical nature, given half a chance, will reestablish itself in a better way. Where the energy is interrupted, I want to hear its stifled cries and tease out the image that binds it. Why has the train stopped at the station and refused to go on? The answers may pop out this moment or elude us for years. We set up a conversation, primitive though our vocabulary may be, a vocabulary of subtle movements to evoke the feeling images stunned into long silence by bodily trauma.

EXERCISE EIGHTY-EIGHT: MOVEMENTS OF PLEASURE

Ask your client to make movements which feel pleasurable to her while you watch and note each action. The client begins with small slow movements and lets these movements expand if it feels right. As she learns to respond to her body from inside, your client develops an individual vocabulary. A sequence of movements might occur like a waking dream, which uncannily leads back to unresolved childhood actions, enacting a forgotten drama. Just as psychic images tumble past our expectation as we recall a dream, so physical movement, when it is initiated inwardly, will follow its own inevitable, integral sequence.

EXERCISE EIGHTY-NINE: ORDINARY GESTURES

As therapists, we need to work with ourselves on a daily basis. I'm sitting in my chair, writing. My neck feels stiff and held, so I move slowly to heighten that feeling before I stretch away from rigid structuring. My right leg is crossed over the left too tightly. I play with a movement in my right leg, a rocking motion with my foot propped against a foot stool, swinging the knee out and back. The purpose is not to create a performance for someone to watch, but to move creatively out of primitive feeling. If we feel pleasure and explore it simply, simple gestures and commonplace tasks will have poetry for us. In this exercise, wherever you are, repeat ordinary gestures and enhance them with greater presence.

EXERCISE NINETY: CORE MOVEMENT

Your client stands alone or with you as witness, and moves only when he feels the movement form within him. Tell your client not to attempt to understand the movements. Kneeling, squatting, sitting or lying on the floor, your client moves in whatever way he is compelled to from within. Remember or take notes of the movements and the feelings and images the dance conveys to you. Share them with the client, who also discusses his experience.

EXERCISE NINETY-ONE: AS A DANCE

Alone or with you as witness, your client explores the following questions through core movement and inner attention. Tell him to express in the form of a dance, (a) his wholeness, (b) his boundaries, (c) his power, (d) his love, (e) his groundedness, (f) his individuality, (g) his devotion, (h) his freedom.

Chapter 39

Dreams and the Body

The adult does not understand symbolism easily, and only occasionally does he succeed in grasping the symbolic connections that some piece of human undertaking has with the unconscious. The child possesses this understanding intuitively, a fact which should be borne in mind in theoretical or practical studies of children. This intuition of the first years of life is quickly lost and replaced by what is usually called common sense, but which in reality is merely stupidity based on repression.

Georg Groddeck, "The Compulsion To Use Symbols"

Recently I have been combing through my journals dating back many years and the most revealing and truthful awareness of my situation day by day has been disclosed through them. In particular one dream announced to my deaf ears the necessity of my terrible reduction. "What will break through this person's intractable character?" the dream asked me. I knew the dream person as an acquaintance and the dream exposed to my amused approval the depth and range of the persons intransigence. "Khartoum" the dream answered. I remembered vaguely that the English were destroyed in battle at Khartoum. At the time of the dream, I did not remotely guess that the dream spoke of my future, predicting a necessarily vast internal upheaval.

Dreams record a path of psychic footprints through emotional flurries, fights with a lover, insoluble dilemmas. They question us

243

about our meaning and surface uncanny revelations of the past, present and future. Dream journals, if studied after a few years, are extraordinarily valuable in disclosing ourselves in our hidden aspect. Dreams dip into the river of images that make up our psychic flow corresponding to the river of energy that enlivens the body-self. As Georg Groddeck has stated, something lives us, dreams us, pumps our blood, directs our steps, communicates with us, chooses our accidents and illnesses and prepares our death. The night dreams and waking fantasies, like our postural attitude, tell us about the myth or story we are living. By attending to the dream and waking fantasy and studying our body's response, we openly engage in dialogue with the it or self that holds the balance of power in our lives. In a mythic and somatic psychology it makes sense for us to study the language of our body and our dreams and walk through our dream stories in the full light of day, so that we have more voice in our own fate.

We do not speak the dream without our voice embracing or disowning our words. Our shoulders rise up in fear and we turn slightly as the dream shifts to another scene. The body struggles with the spoken dream wrapping itself around the drama, resisting and revealing the hidden content through subtle gestures. At times the dream speaks through us as if our conscious life were mere tissue paper. Our body opens to its unconscious expression. For a moment our character relaxes its grip. We are reminded of our profound freedom in life. Our sense of imprisonment is a sham.

Sometimes the dreamer is humble before a voice that instructs and warns as a powerful teacher. Occasionally a dream captures us, both the client and therapist, binding us to a common mythology, calling us away from separateness. Always the dream bears down upon us with its force, and our bodies play out our responses through impulse and defense. Exploring the body of the dream brings together powerful techniques, otherwise held separate, that clarify our unconscious life. The following paragraphs describe a variety of ways to explore dreams, processes that can be interrupted when appropriate to investigate our bodily response.

EXERCISE NINETY-TWO: TELL THE DREAM

Ask your client to tell her dream. Sometimes, it is best simply to leave the dream alone. It is enough to hear the dream, to be a witness to it. Dreams often should not be interrupted. They are their own best statement as symbols that need no translation and their being told is powerful and sufficient. Sometimes the dreamer, eager for comment, does better by sitting with the images awhile.

EXERCISE NINETY-THREE: PAINT THE IMAGE

Suggest that your client explore the images by painting or drawing them. The act of painting and drawing connect the dreamer directly to the unconscious origins of the dream image and brings forth surprising compliments to the original dream statement. The client may experience painting as both an unconscious and conscious process.

EXERCISE NINETY-FOUR: WALKING THROUGH

After the dreamer tells the dream, have him stand and walk through the dream repeating it a second time. Stop the recounting from time to time to ask for further detail. The dreamer imagines the scene spatially, and the dream, no longer merely dramatic, becomes a drama. As the client gains spatial awareness, the dream extends past the blind voice dependent on sequence. Envisioned, the dream comes upon him all at once. Once the dramatic embodiment of the dream takes place by the client's walking through it, a range of possible actions presents themselves. Have your client report his experience, and share with him your impressions.

EXERCISE NINETY-FIVE: OBSERVING POSTURAL SET

As your client walks through the dream, notice her physical relationship to the dream material. Perhaps her posture is characterological and represents no change from day to day existence, but the dream provides a vital context to work with the hunched or elevated shoulders, the stoic facial mask or the unprotected child stance. By changing the postural set, your client shifts her emotional attitude to the dream. Then ask her to walk through the dream once more. Sometimes the dream activity provokes a bodily response which can be explored. Observe how your client breathes or holds her breath. In what way does her body open to the dream? In what way does her body defend against the dream?

EXERCISE NINETY-SIX: IN TRANCE

The dream-telling process often induces a trancelike state which allows the dreamer greater access to unconscious material. You can talk to the unconscious as a healing process or ask questions while watching the body's response. The trance can be deepened by attention to grounding or listening to the breath. If you are trained in hypnosis and trancework, you can deepen trance by prescribing a physical ritual. An example could be: "Walk in a circle as if descending circular stairs clockwise. When you reach the next floor below, tell me what you notice." Remember to have your client reverse the process and ascend the stairs in a counterclockwise direction at the end of the exercise.

EXERCISE NINETY-SEVEN: GESTALT

Sometimes the dream reveals itself when the client becomes some aspect of the environment—the earth, sky, air, bush, any inanimate object—and speaks for these elements as if they have consciousness. The client can assume the identity of participants in the dream as well, on the principle that all aspects of the dream represent us. Ask your client to speak as if she were the sky in her dream. Explore with her the different roles she may play out in the dream.

In a dream in which the dream figure is severely frightened by towering waves, the dreamer experiences an exhilarating freedom from burden and fear when identified with the sky. The dreamer is thus able to integrate the emotionally detached sky and her fear, the latter becoming less overwhelming and consequently more bearable.

EXERCISE NINETY-EIGHT: TAKING PARTS

The therapist takes a part in the dream and re-enacts the dream with the dreamer. For example, the dreamer finds herself enraged by a conversation with her dutiful, compliant mother. Her brother stands idly by, fooling with the handle of an oven door which breaks off. The oven enlarges suddenly becoming a gaping hole as she awakens. The dreamer chooses the role of her mother. The therapist plays the brother, who the client strongly identifies with as being in a posture of passive rebellion. You allow the dream drama to capture you and your client in its emotional grip. Observe how your client responds to you. Notice how you feel as the rebellious brother. Discuss your feelings with your client and ask your client for her experience during the dream drama.

EXERCISE NINETY-NINE: DIALOGUE

As you play out the dream, stop the scene and extend the dialogue, or question the "players" about their feelings. Concerning the previous dream, you might ask, "How do you feel when the mother looks at you with cow-like eyes?" "Oven, why have you grown so large?"

EXERCISE ONE HUNDRED: REWRITE

As a drama you can rewrite scenes and change endings. You can act out several endings. Have your client rewrite his dream with a different ending. In one drama the dreamer had her dead father return. When the client played her mother in this dream, she sobbed spontaneously. The lethargy that previously dominated the dream released in tears and was understood later as unexpressed and unresolved grief.

Embodied dreamwork fills out the dream with our physical engagement. An older woman client dreamed of a lover who met her in a beautiful old mansion that had been converted into a hotel. He wined and dined her. They danced into the evening and eventually he escorted her into an elegant bedroom. As they embraced tenderly, he attempted to kill her by strangling her. She awoke in shock. She had no idea what the dream meant. As she walked through the living drama of the dream, I instructed her to ask the following questions. "Why are you in the dream?"

"I have a message for you," the lover responded.

"Why did you strangle me?"

"To get your attention."

"Couldn't you just have told me the message?"

"You don't listen." The lover told her the message. When she sat down breaking the trance, she could not remember the dialogue. Over and over I read her the dialogue we had just witnessed. The dream spoke eloquently to her resistance in therapy and her life. It was very hard for her to remember from week to week what had happened in her therapy. The dream became a touchstone, reminding her of her life-denying stance.

Once clients learn a respectful and receptive style of working with dreams, I draw on their own wisdom and instincts to interpret and respond to the images. Often a dream takes us both over as it enacts itself through us. The dream has a numinosity and becomes an invitation to the self.

Chapter 40

Conclusion:
Character and Myth

In short, myths describe the various and sometimes dramatic breakthroughs of the sacred (or the "supernatural") into the World. It is this sudden breakthrough of the sacred that really establishes the World and makes it what it is today. Furthermore, it is as a result of the intervention of Supernatural Beings that man himself is what he is today, a mortal, sexed, and cultural being.

Mircea Eliade, *Myth and Reality*

Therapeutic systems do not heal. They set the rules for the therapist-client interaction and direct our expectations through a model of wholeness. In a psychological body therapy we have conceptual structures that define our work, and key words that are understood across the wide spectrum of the bodywork field such as: grounding, boundaries, breath, energy, emotional expression, catharsis, kinesthetic awareness, splitting, character armor, Reich's seven segments, hyper- and hypotense muscle. But these, powerful tools that they are, are not what heals.

I have in this book attempted to describe the basic metaphors of a psychological bodywork in the context of a wider psychology. In bodywork we need not tolerate a narrow vision of our humanity. Our inclusive theory is interpersonal and intrapsychic, mythic as well as somatic. It draws from drive and ego, from self and somatic psychologies. Outside the bodywork field, there are practitioners we learn from like Winnicott and Jung whose sophisti-

249

cated concept of humanity never excluded the body in therapy. There are others like Klein and Kohut whose work enriches us all.

From a broad perspective, the commitment to psychology as a science should not blind us to psychology as a healing myth. Psychology not only describes behavioral patterns but exercises the imagination. It asks questions that literary and religious minds have sought answers to, questions concerning the nature of humanity, questions concerning our fate as sentient beings in a nonhuman world. Psychology provides a mirror with language to observe our experience and interpret our inner guardians of light and darkness. Clients in search of meaning find in the continuity of psychological teaching a comforting and instructive story that as myth teaches us our place in the world.

Freud was not content to passively identify with the myth of Oedipus. He wrote a myth about the primal horde and he shaped the stories of Moses to his own purposes. Clients often come to us having lost faith in themselves and in the direction of their life. They seek a new way to understand themselves. With myth, we must walk lightly and not persuade. We must, as therapists, be careful that insight does not freeze into doctrine and that our voice does not become strident with persuasive argument. Myth finds us when we open ourselves to life. Our healing is not with theory but through the awakening energetic life within our body selves.

When Jung asked himself what myth he was living during the year following his break-up with Freud, he found he was struggling against autonomous elements of self threatening the dissolution of his ego. He could not afford to hold onto meaningless fictions about his life. He sought out a mythology that contained and expressed him, a mythology that might organize his disparate being around a deeper more compelling self that endures. He developed an immediate, personal mythology from dreams and visions. Although raised as a Protestant, Jung found vision and integration through the myth of Faust and the language of alchemy. Reich, on the other hand, appears in his last years to have taken comfort in the Christ myth that explained the suffering he experienced at the hands of the world.

Character represents a conversion at the hand of man (or woman), our own hand, a house built on the sands of dissociation rather than the rock of a durable and functional self. Ego-centered conversion experiences gives the illusion of wholeness by excluding aspects of our nature, our sexuality, our aggression and our desperate need. Through denial, we can imagine that evil takes place out there while we remain pure. Mythic conversion experiences at the hand of God, such as St. Paul describes, can heal profound injuries, because myth is a creation drama in which a new reality comes into being out of the deepest levels of self and the actors are supernatural beings. That sacred nature stands up in us and throws off the dark net of our despairing ways.

As psychological body therapists our task is not to address character in isolation, but rather in relationship to the core self, which becomes personified in the divine child and the hero and heroine in mythology. The core self slays the dragon. It lies partially hidden as potential in the vital body of our imaginative being and finds voice in dreams and myth. Our clients attune to their potential nature by feeling the connection of their spine, pelvis and legs. Bodywork touches off images and dreams. As clients throw off the heavy character armor and draw together what was lost in themselves, they may instinctively toss a light mythic cloak around their shoulders for protection.

Character is a necessary binding fiction in the face of splitting. A mythology of our own provides a flexible, expansive alternative to character. Our integrated self needs room to be discontinuous. Separateness and differentiation in our nature allows for creativity and surprise. We do not thrive as a living body contracted fearfully toward its center. Character contracts; myth expands. Character closes down on anxiety while myth opens to pain and pleasure, adventure and awareness. Indeed, it sometimes happens that when we no longer hide from the storm, we are driven for a time by fierce winds into strange and miraculous seas.

Myth, not character, reveals our true nature. Myth is the language of the unconscious and character the defense of the ego. Myth is the sail that holds the winds of spirit propelling us through the natural and archetypal world. The lush poetry of the human spirit has left us many alternatives. We can be gathered up by the intellectual serenity of Apollo who saw our fleeting humanity like so many leaves falling from a tree, or be guided by Hermes, an unlikely youth with the down of puberty still on his upper lip. In our transforming terror, Hermes may look like the devil as we integrate our dark side, our shadow. We can survive the anguish of the cross of Christ and be lifted up in the living body that does not die; or like David in victory, we can dance naked in Jerusalem in ecstatic surrender to God.

Systems never heal. The therapeutic mask of healer accomplishes no cure. Only the living body, our inspired nature, touches deeply enough to awaken the power of life in others. Over time our voice embodies. It is likely that we pay a high price to speak from a grounded place. Therapists who put their foot upon the path of healing do so consciously—or unconsciously—to heal themselves. They step with easy footing upon a quiet grassy path and the cool breeze of the mountains playfully tugging at their hat. Years later they find themselves desolate in a treacherous swamp with little idea of their path in or out. At such times the therapist is called upon to find that divine nature within the self that can light a fire to keep him warm for the night and the many nights to come.

Many of us have been well-intentioned healers only wishing to help other people, blind to our own precarious footing. It was inevitable that we should be led by the flickering lights into the depths of the swamp. Among our teachers, there are clients that reveal mysteries from the depths of their being. They call us away from the safety of superficiality and shallowness of feeling. They call us out of our intellectual reverie, our egocentricity and our professional persona into dangerous and essential places.

And there are always clients who, out of desperate pain, will stalk our unconscious seeking companionship with us through the doorway of our deepest injury. They have looked through the windows of our parked car more than once. They will reduce us. They will call us down from our imagined therapeutic height out of envy, rage or rejected love. Experienced therapists have learned much about themselves not only from their teachers and therapists, but also from their clients, surrendering to the truth and suffering the death of ego. But such deaths are part of our individuation as we integrate the lost worlds of self rudely brought to our notice by clients, lovers and friends. Usually our enemies, if we have any, do not know us well enough to strike so deeply.

Psychological and somatic insights are bought with a price. The theorists have searched their own nature and been instructed by humiliating defeats. They have exposed their vulnerabilities through their writings. Psychology is a sharp sword indeed, established by Freud on the uncompromised truth about ourselves, relative as that might be. Our bodies cannot be left out of the sacred circle of our humanity. Our bodies expose and uplift us. Our bodies can lead us to the deep understanding of spiritual embodiment. Embodiment as wholeness is not homogenous like a rubber ball, but is a multiplicity of natures, like the planet earth with divergent peoples bathed by the same oceans, breathing the same air where relatedness does not depend on agreement. Through embodiment and through the development of a functional and a durable self, we draw the high energies to us and hold to an earth, ocean and sky that fills out our human nature.

divine.

Bibliography

Abel, Donald C. *Freud: On Instinct and Morality.* Albany: State University of New York Press, 1989.

Arlow, Jacob A. and Charles Brenner. *Psychoanalytic Concepts and the Structural Theory.* New York: International University Press, 1964.

Balint, Michael. *Primary Love and Psycho-Analytic Technique.* New York: Liveright Publishers, 1965.

Bettelheim, Bruno. *Freud and Man's Soul.* New York: Random House, 1984.

———. *Freud's Vienna and Other Essays.* New York: Alfred A. Knopf, 1990.

Blake, William. *Poems and Letters.* Ed. J. Bronowski. Middlesex, England: Penquin, 1986.

Blanck, Gertrude and Rubin Blanck. *Ego Psychology: Theory and Practice.* New York: Columbia University Press, 1974.

———. *Ego Psychology II: Psychoanalytic Developmental Psychology.* New York: Columbia University Press, 1979.

Boadella, David, ed. *Energy and Character: The Journal of Bioenergetic Research.* Abbotsbury, Weymouth, Dorset, England: Abbotsbury Publishers.

Brenner, Charles. *An Elementary Textbook of Psycho-Analysis.* Garden City, New York: Doubleday Anchor books, 1957.

———. *Psychoanalytic Technique and Psychic Conflict.* New York: International University Press, 1976.

Brome, Vincent. *Ernest Jones: Freud's Alter Ego.* New York: W. W. Norton, 1983.

———. *Freud and his Early Circle.* New York: William Morrow and Co., 1967.

———. *Jung: Man and Myth.* New York: Atheneum, 1978.

Buckley, Peter, ed. *Essential Papers on Object Relations.* New York: New York University Press, 1986.

Carotenuto, Aldo. *A Secret Symmetry: Sabina Spielrein Between Jung and Freud.* Trans. Arno Pomerans, John Shepley, and Krishna Winston. New York: Pantheon. 1982.

Chasseguet-Smirgel, Janine. *The Ego Ideal: A Psychoanalytic Essay on the Malady of the Ideal.* Trans. Paul Barrows. New York: W. W. Norton, 1984.

———, and Bela Grunberger. *Freud or Reich? Psychoanalysis and Illusion.* Trans. Claire Pajaczkowska. New Haven: Yale University Press, 1986.

Coles, Robert. *Anna Freud: The Dream of Psychoanalysis.* New York: Addison-Wesley Publishers, 1992.

Davis, Madeleine and David Wallbridge. *Boundary and Space: an Introduction to the Work of D. W. Winnicott.* New York: Brunner/Mazel Publishers, 1981.

Decker, Hannah S. *Freud, Dora, and Vienna, 1900.* New York: Macmillan Company, 1991.

Deutsch, Helene. *Neuroses and Character types: Clinical Psychoanalytic Studies.* Ed. John D. Sutherland. Trans. W. D. Robson-Scott. New York: International University Press, 1965.

———. *Psycho-Analysis of the Neuroses.* London: The Hogarth Press, 1951.

Donn, Linda. *Freud and Jung: Years of Friendship, Years of Loss.* New York: Charles Scribner's Sons, 1988.

Eliade, Mircea. *The Forge and the Crucible.* Trans. Stephen Corrin. Chicago: The University of Chicago Press, 1978.

———.*Myth and Reality.* Trans. Willard R. Trask, New York: Harper and Row, 1975.

Esman, Aaron H., ed. *Essential Papers on Transference.* New York: New York University Press, 1990.

Fairbairn, W. Ronald D. *Psychoanalytic Studies of the Personality.* London: Tavistock Publishers, 1966.

Feldenkrais, Moshe. *Awareness Through Movement: Health Exercises for Personal Growth.* New York: Harper and Row, 1977.

Ferenczi, Sandor. *The Clinical Diary of Sandor Ferenczi.* Ed. Judith Dupont. Trans. Michael Balint and Nicola Zardoy Jackson. Cambridge: Harvard University Press, 1988.

Ferenczi, Sandor and Otto Rank. *The Development of Psychoanalysis*. Ed. George H. Pollack. Trans. Caroline Newton. Chicago: Chicago Institute for Psychoanalysis, 1986.

Fine, Reuben. *The History of Psychoanalysis: New Expanded Edition*. Northvale, New Jersey: Jason Aronson, 1990.

Foucault, Michel. *Mental Illness and Psychology*. Trans. Alan Sheridan. New York: Harper and Row, 1976.

Freeman, Lucy. *The Story of Anna O*. New York: Walker and Co., 1972.

Freud, Sigmund. *The Complete Letters of Sigmund Freud to Wilhelm Fliess, 1887–1904*. Trans. and ed. Jeffrey Moussaieff Masson. Cambridge: Harvard University Press, 1985.

————and Ernest Jones. *The Complete Correspondence of Sigmund Freud and Ernest Jones, 1908–1939*. Ed. R. Andrew Paskauskas. Cambridge: Harvard University Press, 1993.

————. *Origins of Psychoanalysis: Letters to Wilhelm Fliess, Drafts and Notes, 1887–1902*. Ed. Marie Bonaparte, Anna Freud, and Ernst Kris. Trans. Eric Mosbacher and James Strachey. New York: Basic Books, 1954.

————. *The Standard Edition of the Complete Psychological Works of Sigmund Freud*. 24 vols. Trans. James Strachey. London: The Hogarth Press, 1975.

Freud, Anna. *The Ego and the Mechanisms of Defense*. New York: International University Press, 1976.

————. *The Psychoanalytical Treatment of Children: Lectures and Essays*. New York: Schocken Books, 1974.

Freud, Martin. *Sigmund Freud: Man and Father*. New York: Jason Aronson, 1983.

Fromm, Erich. *Greatness and Limitations of Freud's Thought*. New York: Harper and Row, 1979.

Fromm-Reichmann, Frieda. *Principles of Intensive Psychotherapy*. Chicago: The University of Chicago Press, 1950.

Gay, Peter. *Freud: A Life For Our Time*. New York: W. W. Norton, 1988.

————. *A Godless Jew: Freud, Atheism, and the Making of Psychoanalysis*. New Haven: Yale University Press, 1987.

Greenberg, Jay R. and Stephen A. Mitchell. *Object Relations in Psychoanalytic Theory.* Cambridge: Harvard University Press, 1983.

Groddeck, Georg. *The Book of the It.* New York: International University Press, 1976.

———. *The Meaning of Illness: Selected Psychoanalytic Writings.* Ed M. Masud R. Khan. Trans. Gertrud Mauder. London: The Hogarth Press, 1977.

Grosskurth, Phyllis. *Melanie Klein: Her World and Her Work.* New York: Alfred A. Knopf, 1986.

———. *The Secret Ring: Freud's Inner Circle and the Politics of Psychoanalysis.* New York: Addison-Wesley Publishers, 1991.

Guntrip, Harry. *Psychoanalytic Theory, Therapy, and the Self: A Basic Guide to the Human Personality in Freud, Erikson, Klein, Sullivan, Fairbairn, Hartmann, Jacobson, and Winnicott.* New York: Basic Books, 1973.

———. *Schizoid Phenomena, Object-Relations and the Self.* Madison, Conn: International University Press, 1989.

Hannah, Barbara. *Jung: His Life and Work-A Biographical Memoir.* New York: Putnam's, 1976.

———. *Encounters with the Soul: Active Imagination as Developed by C. G. Jung.* Santa Monica: Sigo Press, 1981.

Herman, Judith Lewis. *Trauma and Recovery.* New York: Basic Books, 1992.

Hillman, James. *Egalitarian Typologies Versus the Perception of the Unique.* Dallas: Spring Publishers, 1980.

Hinshelwood, R. D. *A Dictionary of Kleinian Thought.* London: Free Association Books, 1991.

Horney, Karen. *Final Lectures.* Ed. Douglas H. Ingram. New York: W. W. Norton, 1987.

Hughes, Judith M. *Reshaping the Psycho-Analytic Domain: The Works of Melanie Klein, W.R.D. Fairbairn, and D. W. Winnicott.* Berkeley: University of California Press, 1989.

Isbister, J. N. *Freud: An Introduction to his Life and Work.* Cambridge, England: Polity Press, 1985.

Jacobi, Jolande. *The Psychology of C. G. Jung: An Introduction with Illustrations.* New Haven: Yale University Press, 1962.

————. *The Way of Individuation.* Trans. R.F.C. Hull. New York: New American Library, 1983.

Jacobson, Edith. *The Self and the Object World.* Madison, Conn: International University Press, 1986.

Jaffe, Aniela. *From the Life and Work of C. G. Jung.* Trans. R.F.C. Hull. New York: Harper and Row, 1971.

————.*Jung's last Years and Other Essays.* Trans. R.F.C. Hull and Murray Stein. Dallas: Spring Publishers, 1984.

————. *Was C. G. Jung a Mystic? and Other Essays.* Ed. Robert Hinshaw. Trans. Diana Dachler and Fiona Cains. Einsiedeln, Switzerland: Daimon Verlag, 1989.

Johnsen, Lillemor. *Integrated Respiration Theory/Therapy: Birth and Rebirth in the Fullness of Time.* (no publisher listed) 1981.

Johnson, Don. *Body.* Boston: Beacon Press, 1983.

Johnson, Stephen M. *Characterological Transformation: the Hard Work Miracle.* New York: W. W. Norton, 1985.

————. *Humanizing the Narcissistic Style.* New York: W. W. Norton, 1987.

Jones, Ernest. *The Life and Work of Sigmund Freud.* 3 vols. New York: Basic Books, 1957.

Juhan, Deane. *Job's Body: A Handbook for Bodywork.* Barrytown, New York: Station Hill Press, 1987.

Jung, C. G. *The Collected Works of C. G. Jung.* 20 vols. Ed. Sir Herbert Read, Michael Fordham, Gerhard Adler, William McGuire Princeton: Princeton University Press, 1953–1979.

————. *Analytical Psychology: Notes of the Seminar Given in 1925 by C. G. Jung.* Ed. William McGuire. Princeton: Princeton University Press, 1989.

————. *C. G. Jung: The Visions Seminars.* 2 vols. Zurich: Spring publications, 1976.

————. *Dream Analysis: Notes of the Seminar Given in 1928–1930, by C. G. Jung.* Ed. William McGuire. Princeton: Princeton University Press, 1984.

————. *Nietzsche's Zarathustra: Notes of the Seminar Given in 1934–1939, by C. G. Jung.* 2 vols. Ed. James L. Jarrett. Princeton: Princeton University Press, 1988.

Keleman, Stanley. *The Human Ground: Sexuality, Self and Survival.* Berkeley: Center Press, 1975.

Kernberg, Otto. *Borderline Conditions and Pathological Narcissism.* New York: Jason Aronson, 1979.

Khan, M. Masud R. *The Privacy of the Self: Papers on Psychoanalytic Theory and Technique.* Madison, Conn: International University Press, 1974.

Klein, Melanie. *The Writings of Melanie Klein.* 4 vols. Ed. Roger Money-Kyrle. New York: Macmillan, Inc., 1975.

———. *The Selected Melanie Klein.* New York: Macmillan, Inc., 1986.

Klein, Melanie and Joan Riviere. *Love, Hate, and Reparation.* New York: W. W. Norton, 1964.

Kohut, Heinz. *The Analysis of the Self: A Systematic Approach to the Psychoanalytic Treatment of Narcissistic Personality Disorders.* New York: International University Press, 1971.

———. *The Restoration of the Self.* New York: International University Press, 1977.

———. *Self Psychology and the Humanities: Reflections on a New Psychoanalytic Approach.* Ed. Charles B. Strozier. New York: W. W. Norton, 1985.

———. *The Kohut Seminars of Self Psychology and Psychotherapy With Adolescents and Young Adults.* Ed. Miriam Elson. New York: W. W. Norton, 1987.

Laplanche, J. and J.-B. Pontalis. *The Language of Psycho-Analysis.* Trans. Donald Nicholson-Smith. New York: W. W. Norton, 1973.

Loewald, Hans W. *Papers on Psycho-Analysis.* New Haven: Yale University Press, 1988.

Lowen, Alexander. *The Betrayal of the Body.* New York: Macmillan, 1967.

———. *Bioenergetics.* New York: Penguin, 1975.

———. *Depression and the Body.* New York: Penguin, 1972.

———. *The Language of the Body.* New York: Macmillan, 1958.

———. *Narcissism: Denial of the True Self.* New York: Macmillan, 1983.

———. *The Way to Vibrant Health: A Manual of Bioenergetic Exercises.* New York: Harper & Row, 1977.

Mahler, Margaret S. *On Human Symbioses and the Vicissitudes of Individuation: Infantile Psychosis.* New York: International University Press, 1978.

——, Fred Pine and Annie Bergman. *The Psychological Birth of the Human Infant: Symbiosis and Individuation.* New York: Basic Books, 1975.

Maidenbaum, Aryeh, and Stephen A. Martin. *Lingering Shadows: Jungians, Freudians, and Anti-Semitism.* Boston: Shambhala, 1991.

Marcus, Steven. *Freud and the Culture of Psychoanalysis: Studies in the Transition from Victorian Humanism to Modernity.* New York: W. W. Norton, 1984.

Masterson, James F. and Ralph Klein ed. *Psychotherapy of the Disorders of the Self: The Masterson Approach.* New York: Brunner/Mazel Publishers, 1989.

McGuire, William, ed. *The Freud/Jung Letters: The Correspondence Between Sigmund Freud and C. G. Jung.* Trans. Ralph Manheim and R.F.C. Hull. Bollingen Series XVII. Princeton: Princeton University Press, 1974.

Miller, Alice. *The Drama of the Gifted Child.* Trans. Ruth Ward. New York: Basic Books, 1981.

Millon, Theodore, *Disorders of Personality D.S.M. III: Axis II.* New York: John Wiley and Sons, 1981.

Myerson, Paul Graves. *Childhood Dialogues and the Lifting of Repression: Character Structure and Psychoanalytic Technique.* New Haven: Yale University Press, 1991.

Neu, Jerome, ed. *The Cambridge Companion to Freud.* Cambridge: Cambridge University Press, 1991.

Neumann, Erich. *Creative Man: Five Essays: Kafka/Trakl/Chagall/Freud/Jung.* Trans. Eugene Rolfe. Bollingen Series LXI, vol. 2. Princeton: Princeton University Press, 1982.

——. "Mystical Man." Trans. Ralph Manheim. *Spring* 1961 (1961): 9–49.

Peters, Uwe Henrik. *Anna Freud: a Life Dedicated to Children.* New York: Schocken Books, 1985.

Phillips, Adam. *Winnicott.* Cambridge: Harvard University Press, 1988.

261

Quinn, Susan. *A Mind of her Own: the Life of Karen Horney.* New York: Summit Books, 1987.

Rank, Otto. *Beyond Psychology.* New York: Dover, 1941.

———. "Der Dopplelganger." *Imago,* 3 (1914): 97–164.

———. *The Double: A Psychoanalytic Study.* Trans. and ed. Harry Tucker, Jr. New York: Meridian, 1971.

Reich, Ilse Ollendorff. *Wilhelm Reich: A Personal Biography.* New York: St. Martin's Press, 1969.

Reich, Peter. *A Book of Dreams.* Greenwich,Ct.: Fawcett,1973

Reich, Wilhelm. *The Bion Experiments on the Origin of Life.* Trans. Derek and Inge Jordan. Ed. Mary Higgins and Chester M. Raphael. New York: Octogon, 1979.

———. *The Cancer Biopathy* (vol.2 of The Discovery of the Orgone). Trans. Andrew White with Mary Higgins and Chester M. Raphael. New York: Farrar, Straus, & Giroux, 1973.

———. *Character Analysis.* 3rd ed. Trans. Theodore P. Wolfe. New York: Farrar, Straus, & Giroux, 1949.

———. *Cosmic Superimposition.* Trans. Mary Boyd Higgins and Therese Pol. New York: Farrar, Straus & Giroux, 1973.

———. *Ether, God, and Devil.* Trans. Mary Boyd Higgins and Therese Pol. New York: Farrar, Straus, & Giroux, 1973.

———. *The Function of the Orgasm.* Trans. Theodore Wolfe. New York: Meridian, 1970.

———. *Genitality in the theory and Therapy of Neurosis.* 2nd ed. Trans. Philip Schmitz. Ed. Mary Higgins and Chester M. Raphael. New York: Farrar, Straus, & Giroux, 1980.

———. *The Impulsive Character and Other Writings.* Trans. Barbara G. Koopman. New York: New American Library, 1974.

———. *Listen, Little Man!* Trans. Ralph Manheim. New York: Farrar, Straus, & Giroux,1974.

———. *The Mass Psychology of Fascism.* Trans. Vincent R. Carfagno. New York: Farrar, Straus, & Giroux, 1970.

———. *The Murder of Christ.* (vol.1 of *The Emotional Plague of Mankind*). New York: Simon and Schuster, 1953.

———. *Passion of Youth: An Autobiography, 1897–1922.* Ed. Mary Boyd Higgins and Chester M. Raphael, with translations by

Philip Schmitz and Jerri Tomkins. New York: Farrar, Straus, & Giroux, 1988.

———. *People in Trouble* (vol. 2 of *The Emotional Plague of Mankind*). New York: Farrar, Straus, & Giroux, 1976.

———. *Reich Speaks of Freud.* New York: Farrar, Straus & Giroux, 1967.

———. *Wilhelm Reich: Early Writings.* Trans. Philip Schmitz. New York: Farrar, Straus,& Giroux, 1975.

Riviere, Joan. *The Inner World and Joan Riviere: Collected Papers, 1920–1958.* Ed Athol Hughes. New York: Karnac Books, 1991.

Roazen, Paul. *Brother Animal: the Story of Freud and Tausk.* New York: New York University Press, 1986.

———. *Freud and His Followers.* New York: Mentor, 1974.

———. *Freud: Political and Social Thought.* New York: Alfred A. Knopf, 1968.

———. *Helene Deutsch: A Psychoanalyst's Life.* Garden City, New York: Anchor Press/Doubleday, 1985.

———. ed. *Sigmund Freud.* Englewood Cliffs, New Jersey: Prentice Hall, 1973.

Rolf, Ida P. *Ida Rolf Talks About Rolfing and Physical Reality.* Ed. Rosemary Feitis. New York: Harper and Row, 1978.

———. *Rolfing: the Integration of Human Structures.* New York: Harper and Row, 1978.

Roustang, Francois. *Dire Mastery: Discipleship from Freud to Lacan.* Trans. Ned Lukacher. Baltimore: John Hopkins University Press, 1982.

Rosenzweig, Saul. *Freud, Jung, and Hall the King-Maker: the Historic Expedition to America (1909) with G. Stanley Hall as Host and William James as Guest.* Kirkland, Wa: Hogrefe and Huber Publishers, 1992.

Ruitenbeek, Hendrik M. *Freud As We Knew Him.* Detroit: Wayne State University Press, 1973.

———. ed. *Heirs to Freud: Essays in Freudian Psychology.* New York: Grove Press, 1967.

Rycroft, Charles. *Anxiety and Neurosis.* London: Maresfield Library, 1988.

St. Clair, Michael. *Object Relations and Self Psychology: An Introduction.* Monterey, Ca: Brooks/Cole Publishers, 1986.

Samuels, Andrew, Bani Shorter and Fred Plant. *A Critical Dictionary of Jungian Analysis.* New York: Routledge and Kegan Paul, 1986.

Sandler, Joseph with Anna Freud. *The Analysis of Defense: The Ego and the Mechanisms of Defense Revisited.* New York: International University Press, 1985.

———. ed. *On Freud's "Analysis Terminable and Interminable."* New Haven: Yale University Press, 1991.

———, Ethel Spector Person, and Peter Fonagy, ed. *Freud's "On Narcissism: an Introduction."* New Haven: Yale University Press, 1991.

———, Christopher Dare, and Alex Holder. *The Patient and the Analyst: the Basis of the Psychoanalytic Process.* New York: International University Press, 1973.

Searles, Harold F. *Collected Papers on Schizophrenia and Related Subjects.* New York: International University Press, 1965.

———. *Countertransference and Related Subjects: Selected Papers.* New York: International University Press, 1979.

———. *My Work with Borderline Patients.* Northvale, New Jersey: Jason Aronson, 1986.

Segal, Hanna. *Introduction to the Work of Melanie Klein.* New York: Basic Books, 1964.

———. *Klein.* London: Karnac Books, 1989. Shapiro, David. Autonomy and Rigid Character. New York: Basic Books, 1981.

———. *Neurotic Styles.* New York: Basic Books, 1965.

Sharaf, Myron. *Fury on Earth: A Biography of Wilhelm Reich.* New York: St. Martin's Press, 1983.

Stanton, Martin. *Sandor Ferenczi: Reconsidering Active Intervention.* Northvale, New Jersey: Jason Aronson, Inc., 1991.

Sterba, Richard F. *Reminiscences of a Viennese Psychoanalyst.* Detroit: Wayne State University Press, 1982.

Stewart, Walter A. *Psychoanalysis: the First Ten Years, 1888–1898.* New York: The Macmillan Company, 1967.

Sulloway, Frank J. *Freud: Biologist of the Mind—Beyond the Psychoanalytic Legend.* New York: Basic Books, 1979.

Svasta, Ed. "Orgasm Reflex: That Elusive Experience." *The Journal of the International Institute for Bioenergetic Analysis.* 5, no. 2 (1993).

Van Der Post, Laurens. "Wilderness—A way of Truth" in *A Testament to the Wilderness.* Ed. Robert Hinshaw. Santa Monica: The Lapis Press, 1985.

Van Herik, Judith. *Freud on Femininity and Faith.* Berkeley: University of California Press, 1985.

Wehr, Gerhard. *Jung: A Biography.* Trans. David M. Weeks. Boston: Shambhala, 1987.

Whitman, Walt. *Leaves of Grass.* New York: New American Library, 1958.

Winnicott, D. W. *The Family and Individual Development.* New York: Routledge, 1989.

———. *Home Is Where We Start From: Essays by a Psychoanalyst.* Ed. Clare Winnicott, Ray Shepherd, and Madeleine Davis. New York: W. W. Norton, 1986.

———. *Human Nature.* New York: Schocken Books, 1988.

———. *The Maturational Precesses and the Facilitating Environment: Studies in the Theory of Emotional Development.* Madison, Conn: International University Press, 1991.

———. *Psycho-Analytic Explorations.* Ed. Clare Winnicott, Ray Shepherd, and Madeleine Davis. Cambridge: Harvard University Press, 1989.

Wolstein, Benjamin, ed. *Essential Papers on Counter-Transference.* New York: New York University Press, 1988.

Yerushalmi, Josef Hayim. *Freud's Moses: Judaism Terminable and Interminable.* New Haven: Yale University Press, 1991.

Young-Bruehl, Elizabeth. *Anna Freud.* New York: Summit Books, 1988.

Zweig, Connie, and Jeremiah Abrams. ed. *Meeting the Shadow: The Hidden Power of the Dark Side of Human Nature.* Los Angeles: Jeremy P. Tarcher, 1991.

Notes

Section I: The Therapist and Transference

Chapter 1: In Search of a Model for Body-Oriented Psychotherapy

1. C. G. Jung, *Memories,Dreams,Reflections,* ed. Aniela Jaffe, trans. Richard Winston and Clara Winston (New York: Random House, 1973), 170.
2. Sigmund Freud, *The Standard Edition of the Complete Psychological Works of Sigmund Freud,* vol. 7, ed. and trans. James Strachey (London: The Hogarth Press, 1975), 284.
3. *Ibid.,* 292.
4. Heinz Kohut, *The Restoration of the Self* (New York: International University Press, 1977), 72.
5. Heinz Kohut,"the Psychoanalyst and the Historian," in *Self Psychology and the Humanities,* ed. Charles B. Stozier (New York: W. W. Norton, 1985), 221–2.
6. *Ibid.,* 221–2.
7. *Ibid.*
8. Georg Groddeck, "Psychic Conditioning and the Psychoanalytic Treatment of Organic Disorders," in *The Meaning of Illness,* ed. by M. Masud R. Khan (London: The Hogarth Press,1977), 116.
9. *Ibid.,* 117.

Section IV: Protest and Emotional Expression

Chapter 19: Protest,Submission, and Surrender

1. Judith Lewis Herman, *Trauma and Recovery* (New York: Basic Books, 1992), 59.
2. *Ibid.*
3. C. G. Jung, *Nietzsche's Zarathustra: Notes of the Seminar Given in 1934–1939 by C. G. Jung,* vol. 2, ed.James Jarrell (Princeton: Princeton University Press, 1988), 972.

Chapter 20: Emotional Expression

1. Wilhelm Reich, *Character Analysis,* trans. Theodore P. Wolfe (New York: Farrar, Straus and Giroux, 1949), 359.
2. *Ibid.,* 358.

Chapter 29: Energetic Release in the Abdomen and Pelvis

1. Ed Svasta,"Orgasm Reflex: That Elusive Experience" in *The Journal of the International Institute for Bioenergetic Analysis,* vol. 5 (Spring 1993): 52–63.

Section V: Embodiment and the Psyche-Soma Correspondence

Chapter 31: The Psyche-Soma Split

1. Sigmund Freud, "Five Lecture on Psychoanalysis," in *S.E.,* vol. 11, 44–5.
2. Sandor Ferenczi, *The Clinical Diary of Sandor Ferenczi,* ed. Judith Dupont, trans. Michael Balint and Nicola Zarday Jackson (Cambridge, Mass.: Harvard University Press, 1988), 170.
3. Heinz Kohut, "The Psychoanalyst and the Historian," in *Self Psychology and the Humanities,* ed. Charles B. Shozier (New York: W. W. Norton, 1985), 218.
4. *Ibid.,* 217.
5. *Ibid.,* 218.

Chapter 34: Six Basic Body Divisions

1. C.G. Jung, *Nietzsche's Zarathustra,* Vol.1, ed. James L. Janett (Princeton, N.J. : Princeton University Press, 1988), 360.
2. Sigmund Freud to Wilhelm Fliess, Vienna, 4 January, 1898, *The Origins of Psycho-analysis: Letters to Wilhelm Fliess, Drafts and Notes: 1887—1902,* ed. Marie Bonaparte, Anna Freud and Ernst Kris (New York: Basic Books, 1954), 242–3.

Chapter 36: Embodiment and Wilderness Man

1. Laurens Van Der Post, "Wilderness-A Way of Truth" in *A Testament to the Wilderness,* ed. Robert Henshaw (Santa Monica, CA: The Lapis Press, 1985), 50.
2. Robert Lawlor, "Dreaming the Beginning," *Parabola* 18, no. 2 (1993): 11–18.

Chapter 37: Character and Uniqueness

1. James Hillman, *Egalitarian Typologies Versus the Perception of the Unique* (Dallas: Spring Publications, 1980), 3.

Index

PRIVATIZING THE PUBLIC SECTOR

How to Shrink Government

E.S. SAVAS

CHATHAM HOUSE PUBLISHERS, INC.
Chatham, New Jersey

PRIVATIZING THE PUBLIC SECTOR
How to Shrink Government

Sponsored by the Manhattan Institute for Policy Research

CHATHAM HOUSE PUBLISHERS, INC.
Post Office Box One
Chatham, New Jersey 07928

PUBLISHER: Edward Artinian
INTERIOR DESIGN: Quentin Fiore
JACKET AND COVER DESIGN: Lawrence Ratzkin
COMPOSITION: Chatham Composer
PRINTING AND BINDING: Hamilton Printing Company

LIBRARY OF CONGRESS CATALOGING IN PUBLICATION DATA

Savas, Emanuel S.
      Privatizing the public sector

      (Chatham House series on change in American
politics)
      Includes bibliographical references and index.
         1. Public Goods.   2. Expenditures, Public.
3. Public Contracts   4. Social institutions.
5. Voluntarism. I. Title.   II. Series.
HB846.5.S26   353'.073   82-4207
ISBN 0-934540-15-2   AACR2
ISBN 0-934540-14-4 (pbk.)

Manufactured in the United States of America

10 9 8 7 6 5 4 3 2 1

To *my wife, Helen, and my sons, Jonathan and Stephen,
with love, for their patience, understanding, and support*

ACKNOWLEDGMENTS

My thanks go to John Diebold, who first set me to thinking about the need for such a book, and to Elinor and Vincent Ostrom, for their stimulating ideas. The Manhattan Institute for Policy Research supported this work, and I'm grateful for it. Most of the typing was done, patiently and well, by Mrs. Blanche Winikoff and Mrs. Daiselle Crawford. Finally, many friends and colleagues in and out of government, too numerous to identify and thank individually, helped provide the experiences and insights that ultimately shaped this book.